CURE
the
CAUSES

Live the Life You Want
Not the One Prescribed

DR. CHRISTINA RAHM

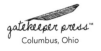
gatekeeper press™
Columbus, Ohio

Cure the Causes: Live the Life you want, not the one prescribed

Published by Gatekeeper Press
2167 Stringtown Rd, Suite 109
Columbus, OH 43123-2989
www.GatekeeperPress.com

ISBN (paperback): 9781662908248
eISBN: 9781662908262

Dedication

THIS BOOK IS dedicated to my children, Duquesne, Preston, Crider, and Merritt Ella for their constant loving encouragement and their constant loving interruptions of my professional and personal life. Without the beautiful chaos of your lives, I would never have been able to do the mission of my life. God has blessed me just by knowing you! I have learned so much from your beautiful hearts. The book is also dedicated to my parents, Stephen Christopher and Jean Rahm, my grandparents, Robert and Lawanda Merritt, Florence Margaret, and James Rahm, and siblings, Mary Margaret and Robert Christopher. I wake up every day thankful for your influence on my life. I praise God for placing you around me, like a blanket in the cold, you have protected me. Thank you for loving me despite my many flaws.

Contents

Foreword

I HAVE A GREAT appreciation for the crew that worked with me to communicate how to get to the root causes of health problems around the world. Together, we can make changes for the betterment of lives and the world. Mary, John, Stephanie, Christopher, Carolyne, Elizabeth, Odessa, Wyeth, Jocelyn, Brad, Patrick, Darren, Robert, Melissa, Jennifer, Clay, Pender, Dino, Dori, Lisa, Mimi, David, Joy, Michael, Crystal, Scott, Henrik, Susan, Bruno, Dani, Temple, Janet, Kristi, Tom, Megan, Viktor, Marihna, Zsuzsa, Dr. Ketskes, Penny, Don, Eric, Lesa, Jessica, Leah, Erin, Jim, Angelica, Nan, Ted, Javier, Laura, Chloe, Preston, Fernando, and the "Wild Ones" from Dexter, Missouri.

Duquesne, Preston, Jean Rahm, Erin, Melissa, Mary, and Mimi Pohlman, thank you for taking extra time on final edits. Special X's and O's to Clay. All of you together, have helped in some way to fulfill getting the need for detoxification and supplementation out into the world.

To my attorneys, I know that most authors do not mention their attorneys but I need to because, without you, I would not have made it. As a little girl growing up in Dexter, Missouri, no one prepared me for a life of war if I decided to do what was right and just. I much prefer peace, but that has not always been my path and I appreciate your dedication to getting the greater knowledge out there and protecting me against those trying to hinder the truth. Females and minorities are often attacked for what they say or believe. Innovative scientists and medical clinical professionals are often criticized or sued for what they know and speak. Thank you for believing in me and for protecting me when I've been attacked for who I am, what I know, and what I have done to bring this knowledge to light. Thank you, Kline, Jeff, Steve, Chris, Phil, and Andy!

To my friends and family, life and people are imperfect, but because of each of you being in my life, the imperfect pieces have become a perfect puzzle. I am so thankful for your beautiful part in all this because without you life would not be nearly as amazing! Peace, love, and happiness- Rahm family, Cook family, Thomas family, Combs family, Merritt family, Holt family, Crider family, Boyd family, and Hayden family.

INTRODUCTION

Cure the Causes

"You are the HELP and the SOLUTION you are searching for."

—*Dr. Christina Rahm*

I DID NOT FEEL like myself. For the past few weeks, I had been feeling dizzy and nauseated. My son was just a few weeks old and his two older brothers were young children, ages five and eight. It didn't even cross my mind that I could be pregnant.

I developed severe pain in my back. At my doctor's insistence, I began undergoing tests that included an MRI. Tests revealed that I had syringomyelia, a disorder in which a cyst, tumor, or cavity form within the spinal cord. Initially, I was in shock. Surgery or radiation was discussed. I underwent two rounds of radioactive nuclear isotopes, a treatment intended to target the tumor.

While recovering from the procedure, I was still feeling the dizziness and nausea that I had been experiencing all along. The thought that I might be pregnant flashed through my mind. Yes, it could be possible. I asked for a pregnancy test and it was positive!

My doctors insisted that I could not sustain the pregnancy. They spoke my worst fears. They told me that my child probably could not survive and that, if she did, she would have an extremely high chance of developing cancer or having a deformity. Furthermore, the doctors warned that delivering a baby while I had syringomyelia would put my own health in jeopardy and could potentially cause paralysis or death. I consulted numerous experts—even a nuclear physicist—and they all said the same thing. I was told that I had to have a medical abortion to save my life. I refused to listen. I was determined to follow a different path . . . to carry my child and give birth to her.

Months later, my beautiful daughter was born healthy and happy. I had refused to follow the advice of all of the specialists and doctors who had all been certain that the outcome of a healthy child was impossible. My traditional medical doctors had prescribed me one life, which was a life where I was to terminate my pregnancy in order to undergo strenuous medical procedures to save my own life. However, I renounced the life I had been prescribed. There was another way. I was determined to prove it, and I did.

Our medical care today can be lifesaving. It can cure diseases that were deadly just a generation ago. But, what if, instead of curing disease and sickness, we could cure their root causes? What if sickness and disease could be avoided all together, or at least minimized?

I decided to write this book to encourage all of us that it is possible to cure the causes. Our world is currently plagued with harmful toxins. Our earth and, therefore, our bodies, need to detoxify. I believe that it is the toxins that are at the root of the disease and sickness we experience. We need to uproot these toxins so that we can live life to the fullest for more years than we can imagine. Noah of the Bible built the ark at the ripe old age of 600. That means, not only did he live to be more than six times our life expectancy of today, but that he was also vital and physically capable. This should reframe our expectations.

Journey with me as I explore the alternatives in healthcare that we have available right at our fingertips today. There is so much more that you can do to live the life you want to and not the one you have been prescribed.

We can CURE THE CAUSES!

CHAPTER ONE

Your body is a city and you are the mayor! How will you run your city?

"The first wealth is health."

—*Ralph Waldo Emerson*

I WANT YOU TO think of your body as a city. The ideal city is developed and clean. Every aspect is maintained and in good order. There is little pollution in the environment and no trash scattered on the streets. The people are friendly and nice. Everyone in the city is safe.

Now, I want you to imagine what could happen to a city without the proper leadership in place and without a good mayor to govern it. Without a good, strong mayor for the city, bad things start to occur. Gangs begin infiltrating the most run-down areas of the city. Crime rates go up and the city's systems are corrupted. As systems within the city start malfunctioning, overall performance declines.

Just as a city can decline without proper leadership, your body can decline if you—the mayor of your body—do not take care of it.

When babies are born, they typically do not have many impurities. Although they may have been pre-exposed to toxic substances in the womb, babies are born relatively pure. As we age, we are more and more exposed to environmental toxins and pollutants. These impurities eventually cause a toxic state. These toxins can act just like the gangs and pollutants that infiltrate a city.

I want you to understand that you have been pre-elected as the "mayor" of your body for your lifetime. You have no contender to compete against, ever. You have full responsibility. Every system reports and listens to you. No harm can come to your body (your city) unless you allow it. You oversee everything happening around you. You are responsible for maintaining order and cleanliness so that the whole atmosphere can be peaceful and systems can perform at their highest levels.

As the mayor of your city, when systems are not performing, you may start trying to fix the problems at the surface level. When you start to investigate solutions, however, you find that "gangs" have been infiltrating slowly and silently with bad intentions. You find that the problem is much deeper than what you have seen on the surface. In fact, a gang might have already strongly rooted itself within your city causing harm to many areas of your body.

In a city, the gang members may not look suspicious, but they are secretly focused on doing illegal things that harm the city. In fact, they are trying to recruit innocent people to join them and be part of their gang. As a result, gang memberships increase rapidly. The good people begin to hide from the gang members as they continue to wreak more and more havoc. Police try to help but they eventually become overpowered by the gang members. If this continues unchecked, law-abiding citizens will not have a place to live.

This same scenario could happen in your body. Abnormal cells, viruses, parasites, bad bacteria, and fungi can act like gang members and infiltrate your body causing negative inflammation. As the abnormal cells recruit more members, your body can become like a city filled with debris. A massive campaign for cleanup must occur.

Your body is made of cells and molecules, just as a city is made of the people and places within it. A cell is the smallest unit of life, popularly known as the building blocks of life. Imagine that the cells in your body are the people in your city and you are their leader. The people take direction from you, but they also talk to each other. The people can influence one another to become like themselves. Good citizens encourage each other to do good things while gang members try to recruit people to help them wreak havoc. This is where the danger—as well as the solution—lies.

In your body, the bad cells literally "talk" to the good cells and say, "Hey, you need to look like me! Life is great with my gang!" Often, the good cells do not understand the danger, so they listen to the bad cells and become like them. This is how gangs of bad cells develop in your body and spread to other areas. This is the very reason why a breast cancer patient may develop lung cancer as well.

The communication between cells takes place silently. There is no indication that this has happened until the "gang" of bad cells has outgrown all the good cells around it and must move to a new area.

There are many toxic substances that we consume or absorb through the environment. These toxins have the potential to turn good cells into bad cells. When this occurs, the bad cells keep growing in number over time causing inflammation and other factors such as epigenetic changes and autoimmune diseases. As a result, a person can develop diseases such as cancer, psoriasis, diabetes, cardiovascular disorders, and/or COPD, to name a few. Science has proven nearly everything from autism to Alzheimer's have many of the same causes.

Cancer is not a disease that usually occurs overnight; it takes a long, long time to develop. Over time, toxins turn good cells into bad cells and then the bad cells continue to talk to each other and make problems worse. If we take a proactive approach, we may be able to avoid the bad cells altogether, or we may be able to lessen their negative effects on our bodies.

This is why I chose to describe the human body to you as a city. I wanted you to see the whole story, the bigger picture. It takes a proactive approach to run a city, or else the bad things take control. If you think you are powerless, let me assure you that, as a human being, you are a miraculous creature and possess a powerhouse of strength to help you deal with hardships.

My work allows me to meet many people through various platforms. When I talk to audiences and clients, I find that most people have no clue how they are being attacked by toxic substances on a daily basis. When I show them the real picture, almost all of them get a sense of panic until I show them the solutions. Most people feel lost and powerless. They can't see a way out. It is hard to find a way out when you are used to walking on the wrong path. You need someone to show you that you are lost and then guide you to the right path. It is my true intention to educate people. I am both an extrovert and an introvert. This means that while I love people, I also love to be alone. In my career as a research scientist, I get to satisfy both sides of my personality to help people. I get to create formulas in labs and I also get to speak publicly to educate and help people.

I don't know your story. I know that life has not been a bed of roses for any of us. The majority of us have seen many rough days in terms of health, finances, kids, spouses, spirituality, and other matters at one time or another. If there has been a time in your life where the world might have seemed lifeless, I want you to know that this has happened to me too. If you are going through a tough period of your life right now, I want to assure you that you will be okay. Don't give up! As a scientific researcher and a psychologist, I know how miraculous the human brain is. Your mind can overcome every challenge in life. You must not consider yourself powerless against these tiny, toxic substances. Doing nothing to find and eliminate toxins from your life is a huge mistake. Through my travels, one of the primary things I teach people is that they need to detox the bad from their lives. Today is the day to start the detoxification process; not tomorrow, not next week . . . today! Let me assure you that you are not powerless against toxins.

I have heard hundreds of stories of parents who have taken the bravest steps to protect their kids and homes. The mama bear protects her cubs and goes to extreme limits to make sure they are safe. The moment she senses danger, she turns into a fearless warrior. In a similar way, you also need to show a "mama bear attitude" to save yourself, your family, and your environment. You need to be fiercely protective of what you put into your body and just as defensive of what happens outside of your body. Courage does not depend on age, gender, race, or economics. We all have the strength and ability to do extraordinary things if we choose.

The toxic substances in our environment are the intruders that are ready to attack and destroy us. Your body is the only place you will live in for your entire lifetime. You take it with you wherever you go. Will you let toxins rob you of your assets and health? Will you wait for help to arrive? Or, will you shoot down the intruders and defend yourself? There are many different scenarios that I can relay as evidence that, if you are determined to do so, you can maintain 100-percent safety of yourself, your family, and your home. The first step is to realize that you are not powerless and helpless. You have the power to protect your own body and to get rid of the bad things that are inside. You also have the power to help others protect their bodies and the environment. You must also understand the vast intelligence of your own body. Miraculously, your body can take care of itself without any help from you. This is great news! However, toxins accumulate over time. They don't naturally leave the body. When this happens, you have to "take the trash out" and detoxify your body. You have to get rid of them. If you do not pay attention, toxins can build up and your body's systems can begin to decline.

Remember, your body is a city and you are the mayor. You are the leader with all-in, absolute power and authority. How are you going to run your city? Several times during my life, I have had to step in and take control of my health. This mindset has empowered me to beat cancer and overcome other health issues. Through it all, I have chosen to be passionate and loving. I never allow hopelessness to take control of MY LIFE. I want to live my whole life as I want to, and I want my kids to take this same approach in their own lives. I want you to do this as well! I want you to take leadership of your body and of your health. There are proactive steps that you can take. You are in the driver's seat when it comes to decisions regarding your own health.

Earlier in this chapter, I explained that when a baby is born, the cells in her body are typically healthy overall despite the pollution they were exposed to in the womb. The healthy cells in her body grow very rapidly. Over time, as she is exposed to toxins, pollutants, and heavy metals, healthy cells can turn into bad cells and start forming gangs. This can become a very negative and dangerous cycle. When a cell turns bad, it uses negative energy and neural transmitters to communicate with good cells and try to turn them into bad ones. We must protect ourselves. We need to look in the mirror and say to ourselves, "I love you." We must fight against the bad things that attack our minds, bodies, and spirits. We must start doing the things to rid the toxins in our body. We have to clean the inside of our bodies, like the outside. We need to start with a clean slate!

Although it is the responsibility of the good cells to stop the bad cells, sometimes, they can get overwhelmed and start to surrender. Sometimes the good cells have no idea what they should do to stop the bad cells from taking over the body. They do not know how to send a "Batman Signal" or call on Wonder Woman for help!

In order to fight the bad cells, YOU need to have the knowledge and understanding of what to do. You must act quickly or there will be collateral damage. You need to implement solutions that will protect the good cells and get rid of the bad cells. You need to make sure your departments of defense are well fortified with tools to support your innate protective mechanisms.

It is important to note here that you need to have solutions that will protect the good cells and get rid of the bad cells. You don't want to use solutions that will kill the good and bad cells at the same time. You have to fight this battle for victory and NOT to destroy everything in your "city." Your job is to detox the really badly unhealthy cells and save those not yet destroyed, then Restore the cells to the beautiful healthy state your body is meant to live in.

When dealing with cancer, chemotherapy is often implemented to destroy the cancerous, bad cells. However, chemotherapy also destroys the good cells. Sometimes, it is necessary, but what if cancer could have been prevented? What if you could have protected the cells against cancer all along by only putting good things into your body while keeping the bad things out? What if you could clean your body, detox your body, restore your cells, and repair your body?

We can all agree on the fact that a nuclear bomb is a horrible thing to use unless there is no choice. It turns a lively city into ashes in an instant and destroys everything. If there are survivors in a nuclear bomb, they are mutilated and may not have a healthy life ever again. It turns the ground into a useless piece of land. Later, children are often born with deformities. For your city, you don't have to push the button to drop a bomb with such an impact. You are in charge and need to find a middle ground with a targeted approach so that you can wipe out the bad cells only and save the good ones. A proactive approach can help prevent cancer in some cases. Your cells are made to kill cancer cells, just as police can kill an armed criminal. They only need to be properly equipped. If it does occur, there are natural alternatives to consider. Take charge and find out as much as you can about the options that you have. Since you are the mayor of your city with absolute power, you are the final decision maker. No Superman or Wonder Woman is coming to save your city. Believe in yourself that YOU ARE THE POWER YOU NEED to get rid of the bad things. Sometimes, solutions are hidden in plain sight. Your body is a great responsibility and you can take care of it by making the right choices for your life. If you know that some of the cells in your body have been behaving badly, it is time to step in and fix things. Find the strength, courage, and the ability to step up and do what needs to be done. You can say, "You know what? I'm in charge here! I'm the mayor and I'm going to get rid of bad things in my city for good. I am going to make my city beautiful!"

So, the first step is to recognize the problems and then develop daily, effective plans to take action and change things. This way, you can have a healthy life for good. Let's put an end to the gang! Let's start with a clean slate!

Your good cells are happy, but they are vulnerable to being influenced by the bad cells if they are not protected. You must win the fight with the help of the good cells versus bas cells.

Unless you equip the good cells with the right weapons, they can't fight the bad cells. Every single good cell is important and needs the right protection. You must realize how important cells are in your body and how you can help detoxify and nourish them. You must revitalize, repair, and restore!

When you are ready to detoxify your body of the bad cells, you then need to prepare the good ones to help in this process. Remember, cells communicate with one another. The good cells need to get ready to talk to the bad cells and convince them to come over to the good side. You can do this by nourishing your body with the right foods and supplements.

You cannot fight against a strong enemy with a weak army. Thus, you have to train your good cells to become stronger while equipping them with the necessary armor to win. At the same time, you must weaken the bad cells by cutting off the supply of further toxic substances.

As you make the good cells stronger, two things will happen. First, the good cells will begin talking to the bad cells with authority and lead them to become good cells. Their message will be, "you need to be like me." When you support your good cells, they will do this, and your health will improve.

If the good cells are strong enough for the fight, they can actually become executioners and begin to kill the bad cells. It's as simple as that! As you feed your body the right things, the stronger, good cells keep taking the bad ones out and will ultimately put an end to the bad gang members in your body. As the gang dies, your city will be restored. Your body will enjoy balance and peace, or what we call homeostasis. Your city will once again be a beautiful place to live. Your city in your body becomes the most desired place in the world to live and the good news is that it is yours. You own it!

The weapons your body needs come through a detox and wellness plan. There are a number of healthy practices and products you can use to detox your body and flush out the toxic substances. Choosing a nuclear bomb like chemotherapy must be a last resort. First, choose detox!

When you choose a plan of action to detox your body, keep this fact in mind and do not go for the one that wipes out the good cells too because such an option is the last resort. In its place, go for a targeted detox plan that does not destroy the good cells, but only cleanses them. Be a responsible mayor of your city. Protect the good neighborhood and the good people, while you destroy the bad. You are already elected and in charge of your city and have the power to make all the decisions. So, make the decisions that can fill your city with positive, powerful things and get rid of the bad gangs and the bad things once and for all. Make your city beautiful! Detox, clean, repair, restore, and revitalize!

Over the years, I have developed and formulated many products specifically to do these positive things in your body. These products can repair the body's systems and promote communication between them while ridding the body of toxins. But, a detox plan is not a one-size-fits-all solution. A detox plan that has worked for you may not be as effective for your friend or relative. We each have a unique body with a unique DNA. So, you cannot expect a plan to work for you just because it worked for your brother or sister. However, the basic approach is the same to stop or minimize the exposure to toxic substances while also taking the already gathered toxins out like trash.

Remember, you are responsible for cleaning your city and keeping it in the best condition where there is no fear of gang attacks and no bad elements hidden somewhere, ready to attack as soon as they get a chance. You have to make sure that you have the best city, and it is possible through the constant detoxification process.

As you remove the toxic waste from your body to start with

a clean slate, you have to make sure to break it apart in the best way possible so that you safely clean and restore your city. Thus, detox must be a personal plan that can be adjusted to fit your lifestyle.

When I was faced with health issues at an early age, I developed a customized, detoxification plan for myself. It was specifically designed to fulfill my nutrition and detoxification requirements. If I ask you to follow my exact plan, it may not be as effective for you as it is for me because you are unique—your city is different. Now, it does not mean that you cannot eat what I do. Of course, we have the same foods and products available to eat. You can eat the same vegetables and fruits as I do. The difference lies in the level of damage that the toxins have done to your body. So, you need to have a customized detox plan for yourself to keep your mind and body healthy and fit.

When you are running your city as the mayor, keep it in mind that you are not in a rat race.

Your goal is to be a part of a world that has tolerance. You are fighting a battle with yourself for the best life possible. You are not competing to win an award for best mayor of the year. Instead, you are working hard for excellence and to empower your city to become the best it can be. This is the very essence of building a great city. When you are good and send positive vibes to others, you will be rewarded with good returns too. This is the approach that completes a detox plan because you develop yourself on the spiritual side as well. A human being is a combination of mind, body, and soul and one missing piece keeps the picture incomplete. Thus, adopt a detoxification plan with physical, mental, emotional, and spiritual aspects because they are interconnected.

We can CURE THE CAUSES!

YOU are the law

YOU are the judge

YOU are the lawyer

YOU are the law enforcer

YOU are the authority

YOU are the motivator

CHAPTER TWO

Everything is connected

"Until man duplicates a blade of grass, nature can laugh at his so-called scientific knowledge.

Remedies from chemicals will never stand in favor compared with the products of nature, the living cell of the plant, the final result of the rays of the sun, the mother of all life."

—T. A. Edison

IN THE FIRST chapter, I introduced you to the concept of toxicity. I let you know that you are the mayor of your own body and have the power to detoxify yourself. Toxins exist within your body and you must make every effort to rid yourself of them. Toxins also exist within our environment. Your body is under attack by these toxins daily. For this reason, you must protect and detoxify your body on a continual basis. It is your job to help the good cells win and change—or get rid of—the bad cells. Silicas, zeolites, silver ions, magnesium, and other vitamins and minerals, if properly developed and utilized, can help with all of this!

The air is a major aspect of our environment and air pollution is a rising threat. The steep growth of the industrial sector in recent decades has contributed to this dangerous situation. Without acknowledging it, we have been driving our planet to destruction. Humankind is severely impacted by this phenomenon, as the number of patients being diagnosed with neurological disorders, autoimmune diseases, and cancers is the highest on record. I believe that the increase of these diagnoses can be linked to the lack of detoxification from our environment.

The air we breathe is the essence that ensures our existence. However, the air is polluted, which means our bodies are, as well. Toxins come from various sources such as manufacturing and even some of the appliances in our homes. Many of these pollutants even come from generations ago. These released toxins affect us negatively and hurt our planet. Ridding the air of these toxins is the key to our health, wellness, and survival. Zeolites, silica, magnesium, and other ingredients can help the land and water and promote detoxification of our food and bodies.

Air pollution has contributed to a rise in global temperature that we could not have imagined fifty years ago. The rise in overall temperature is causing damage to two shields that protect our environment, which is polar ice and the ozone layer. Polar ice is, in fact, a frozen ocean. It covers the northern and southern regions—the Arctic and Antarctic regions— of our planet. The rise in global temperature is causing these ice caps to melt at an exceedingly alarming rate. This has the potential to disrupt the entire balance of nature.

Polar ice is a reason why our planet's temperature has been stable for millions of years.

These snow-covered regions reflect an enormous amount of light back to space, and this process maintains the overall temperature of planet earth. If these ice caps were completely eradicated, then the overall temperature would rise to an extent where life on earth could be tremendously jeopardized.

The ozone layer is a protective layer around our earth that protects it from harmful radiation emitted by the sun. The ozone layer traps the sun's harmful rays and filters the light. The erosion of the ozone layer has allowed harmful radiation to pierce our atmosphere and further contribute to the rise in global temperature. This has also increased the occurrence of various kinds of skin-related and cancer-causing toxins that affect our minds and bodies.

Appliances such as refrigerators, air conditioners, and microwaves release a great number of greenhouse gases, or chlorofluorocarbons (CFCs), into our environment. The presence of these gases is one reason for the rise in the temperature of our earth and for the depletion of the ozone layer. Without our natural, protective shield, the battle against global warming is even more difficult. We worry about chemicals damaging the globe, yet disregard the damage done to our bodies. We need to wake up!

Air pollution can't be solved instantly, but by taking a few basic steps we can affect positive change. For instance, if more people were to quit smoking, we would see a significant reduction in air pollution as both firsthand and secondhand smoke are very toxic. It is critical to eliminate both from your life. Smoking not only causes harm to the smoker's own body, but it also harms the people around them by polluting the air. Researchers believe that smoking is among the top five causes of air pollution. This is one of the simplest steps to take to detoxify the body and environment.

You can also take care to choose heating, cooling, cooking, and electrical appliances that do not contribute to air pollution. Research items before you make a purchase. What is in your home impacts you and your family daily as well as the environment.

We can also utilize the help of filters that trees provide, which have been gifted to us by nature. Trees have a very specific job of purifying our air by taking in the carbon dioxide (CO_2) and releasing pure oxygen. We should all take up the practice of planting as many trees as possible. You can start by planting a couple of trees in your backyard. You can also encourage your community to plant trees in parks and school playgrounds. This would also promote awareness of the importance of trees among our children. Children imitate what adults do, so we must show them how to care for our planet. One day, our children will take on the responsibility of caring for the environment.

I grew up surrounded by trees, in the small town of Dexter, Missouri. I learned to love them.

I climbed them and hid from my mother at the top of them. I spent countless, wonderful hours sitting in my treehouse that was built in a huge tree by my Grandpa Merritt.

Today, thankfully, there seems to be an increased awareness of the importance of trees. For a time, the rise in cutting down trees just for the sake of urbanization was very alarming. Now, most countries have restricted deforestation as we have begun to realize the importance of trees for the survival of our planet. The International Science and Nutrition Society (ISNS), for which I am honored to serve as Chairman of the Board, is a global organization dedicated to sharing information, understanding data on the science, and living harmoniously with nature. We can all support such organizations. www.sciencenutritionsociety.com

For indoor air, we can choose air filters that can serve the same purpose in our homes that trees do in nature. The World Health Organization (WHO) has stressed the importance of the air inside our homes. Do everything you can to make sure the air inside your home is clean.

We all need to be more aware of the damages of air pollution. We need to be even more aware of the solutions for addressing it. Detoxification has become a necessity today. Our health and our world depend on the layout that Nature has created for us. Pollution and toxins and their impact on polar ice and the ozone layer can be alarming. Toxic waste and the manufacturing of many products with toxic materials have compounded the effects of the existing toxins within our environment. While we can't necessarily control this, we can investigate our lives and take responsibility for what we can change.

Before we move on to the next chapter, I want to address another component, which is spirituality. Detoxification is not just about eliminating spiritual toxins from your body and your environment. It is also about eliminating spiritual toxins. Our lives have physical, mental, and emotional components. We must detoxify mentally, emotionally, and physically while we try to clean the air, land, and water that surrounds us. If we aren't spiritually healthy, we cannot stay physically healthy.

As I said in the previous chapter, the human body is like a city with the person within it as its mayor. This is something more than just a sentence. Every city needs cleansing, just as your body does. However, your body not only needs physical cleansing but mental cleansing as well. A person's thoughts reflect his or her personality. Everything is connected.

This concept applies to our planet as well. As it is essential for a person to have a clean spirit, it is also essential for our planet to have a clean atmosphere. The atmosphere of our planet is, in essence, its spirituality. In this case, however, the toxins that affect our planet's spirituality are indeed us as its inhabitants.

We have diminished the spirit of our planet to an extent where chances of its detoxification require immediate action.

Our planet earth has been in a declining phase since we began utilizing its resources without considering the aftermath. Thus, we have been destroying our planet's very spirit by meaningless spillage of waste, exposure to toxic gases, and depletion of resources. These actions have led to the toxicity of our planet's spirit. The outcome is a polluted atmosphere for us and for our children.

Our planet's spirit is broken. That is why we are tangled in various kinds of diseases and viruses. With a toxic environment surrounding us, all of these circumstances are expected. We must all seriously consider our lifestyles. The lack of physicality due to the abundance of appliances and technical gadgets that make daily tasks "easy" for us is part of the problem.

Decades ago, when the success of our daily tasks was dependent only on human effort, we were all healthier and the occurrence of disease was much less. So many inventions for our modern world provide another way of eliminating physical effort. The lack of physicality has reduced our motivation. We lack the motivation to cleanse ourselves and hence our environment. It may take decades to successfully cleanse and detoxify our planet and fully revive its spirit. We need to cleanse our individual spirits and find the motivation to make this process happen. We have an innate sense of responsibility to detoxify our global atmosphere.

It is our calling to pave the way for future generations to be born into a world where the air is free of toxins and people are free of toxic spirits. This is the kind of world we ought to leave for our children to inherit; a world that is rushing toward peace and prosperity.

We can CURE THE CAUSES!

DETOXIFY

mentally, emotionally,
and physically

CLEAN

the air, land, and water

CHAPTER THREE

Spiritual detoxification

'No two leaves are alike, and yet there is no antagonism between them or between the branches on which they grow.'

—*Mahatma Gandhi*

I MAGINE FOR A moment that you are in a place of darkness—a sea of blackness. You can see a small light, but you don't know how to move toward it. Everything around you is chaos. You can't focus. You feel hopeless. You are bogged down with a sense of overwhelm.

This is spiritual toxicity and it is a reality in our world.

Spiritual toxicity begins in seemingly small ways. Toxins that affect us spiritually include negativity, self-criticism, criticism of others, and unhealthy relationships, among many others. Over time, the effects of these toxins can be devastating. If you do not take steps to remove these toxins along the way, you can end up spiritually toxic.

I cannot stress enough the importance of spiritual detoxification. Pollution and toxins are not just related to our world or our bodies. I believe that pollution can be found within the human spirit. Therefore, detoxification is a process that requires all parts of yourself and all areas of your life. There is no exception; every aspect of your life must be included. Your life has physical, mental, emotional, and spiritual components. Each of us is driven by the traits of our personality. Some people believe that personality is mostly genetic. I believe that environmental factors are much more important in determining personality. When spiritual toxins are in your environment, your mind is impacted in a negative way.

The people you surround yourself with impact your personality and actions. There are people who have toxic personalities and they can impact others in very negative ways. Just as cancer can kill a person physically, toxic people can be cancerous to the human spirit.

You must remove toxic people from your life. Stay away from them. Don't allow yourself to be surrounded by gossip, chaos, and negative thinking. If it is there, then clean it up. Take the negative relationships out, just like you take the trash out to the curb. Use boundaries and eliminate them from your life. Spiritual toxicity will rob you of the joy in your life. It is normal to experience jealousy, self-loathing, envy, or lust at times. However, you must not let such experiences become permanently embedded in your personality. It is easy to see these traits in others, but you must have the courage to be introspective and see them in yourself. Focus on being the best, kindest, nicest, smartest, and most beautiful "you."

I often meet people who share some of their personal issues with me. They share that they are experiencing negativity in their life. Sometimes, it hits me that part of the reason they are stuck in a negative place is that they don't want to change. They don't want to get rid of the negativity in their life so that they can be free to live a life of joy and happiness. I have been in this situation myself. It isn't good. Trust me, do not delay in ridding your life of toxins. I, personally, have made unhealthy decisions at times. Finally, in 2020, I was able to take a leap of faith and rid myself of the negative influences in my personal and professional life. It is scary and hard to take off the band-aid and leave a career or personal relationship that is toxic and negative. Often, the relationships will fight to hold on even when you try to leave. Stay strong. You can weather the storm. There will be sunshine on the other side!

Your thoughts and actions have a serious impact on your spirituality. It is critical to focus on the good, positive thoughts. Instead of focusing on "what if it didn't", rather, think "what if I did?" Optimism is the best remedy for spiritual toxicity. If you begin looking at the brighter side of a situation or decision, you will witness an increase in self-confidence and the outcome will be amazing! For example, when I go into dangerous countries, I think of the great people I will meet and not of all the possible dangers. I surround myself with positive thoughts and energy. You can do the same in any situation. Trust me. I have been through many negative environments and situations, I am still here and you will be too. Don't give up!

There are others who can help you in your quest for spiritual detoxification. Learn to identify the people in your life who can lift you up, encourage you, and tell you the important truths about you. These are people you will need along your journey. You cannot rely solely on yourself during this process. If you do, you will end up being disappointed in yourself and others.

The detoxification process will be an erratic roller coaster, just as life can sometimes be. It is not wise to expect a smooth ride. There will be moments when you feel you could touch the sky. When that happens, embrace it! Reach out and touch the sky! Then, take a moment to acknowledge that you are there because of yourself and others who have helped you along the way. Be humble. Be confident. Be yourself! Then, remember, the more you receive, the more you can give back. You must fill your cup up before you can fill someone else's glass.

Things may not always turn out as you have expected them to. When disappointments come, remain positive in your thinking. You may feel like you have failed. However, you must keep in mind that failure only happens when you give up. In order to spiritually detoxify yourself, you need to pierce out of the cocoon where you are hiding from personal disappointments and stand up to give life another chance. That's what life is all about. It's about fighting a different battle on a different field every single day.

In order for our spiritual lives to evolve and become healthier, it is essential to recognize the essence of life. Disappointment, jealousy, and envy are all toxins that build a sense of self- doubt and self-pity. Those negative energies will spawn hatred. The consequence of allowing hatred into your life is spiritual toxicity. While positive spirituality can have very positive effects for yourself and those around you, negative spirituality, in contrast, has harrowing effects.

People who are suffering from spiritual toxicity may not realize their own state of being. I would suggest that most criminals, who have committed a horrible crime, have done so from a spiritually toxic state. Our spirit decides the course of action we should take. A pure spirit is essential for a healthy and positive lifestyle. In our world today, there is more suicide and homicide than ever. Why? The answer is simple; more people are suffering from spiritual toxicity. You are different. You don't have to keep suffering. The answers are inside you.

At the beginning of this chapter, I asked you to imagine a place of darkness and spiritual toxicity. Now, I want you to imagine that you are soaring high in the sky. You are surrounded by light and warmth. Your mind is clear, and you feel like you can do anything! This is the feeling of being spiritually free.

Do whatever you have to do to detoxify yourself spiritually so that you can live your best life. Although much easier said than done, don't worry what others think. This is about YOU!

A pure spirit is exceedingly essential for a healthy and positive lifestyle.

We can CURE THE CAUSES!

DETOXIFY

Yourself, Your home, Your environment

CHAPTER FOUR

Live the life you want and not the life someone has prescribed

"He who has health has hope, and he who has hope has everything."

—*Arabian Proverb*

I AM GOING TO make a bold statement. The US is turning into a nation of heavy drug users. Let me present two alarming statistics. In 2010, the total expenditure worldwide on pharmaceuticals was $887 billion. By 2022, that number is estimated to reach more than $1.4 trillion.

According to the US Centers for Disease Control and Prevention (CDC), cigarette smoking is the leading cause of preventable disease and death in the United States, accounting for more than 480,000 deaths every year, or about 1 in 5 deaths.

These statistics are great news for the pharmaceutical industry, but they present a huge red flag for the average person. Statistically, there are more and more patients dependent on pharmaceuticals than ever before and that number is expected to increase drastically in just a few short years.

Mahatma Gandhi defined what is most important and worthy of our ambition when he said, "It is health that is real wealth and not pieces of gold and silver." As a scientist and wellness practitioner, I see the relationship between people and pharmaceuticals as an indication of our attitudes about health. To me, they indicate indifference and a careless attitude regarding healthy changes in lifestyle that need to be made. I fear the days when we will not be able to move without popping a few pills. I fully understand and support medical advancements in pharmaceuticals and biotechnology, but they should only be used when a patient does not have another option. They should not be misused! The statistics terrify me. What days are ahead of us? I believe that pharmaceuticals have a place and can certainly help some people live better lives. However, they are overused in our healthcare system today.

How do you feel when someone tells you what to do? If you are like me, you have very little tolerance for someone else trying to dictate your life. Being told what to do is extremely irritating for most people. Human nature makes us want to do just the opposite of what someone tells us to do. Why is it that we allow the pharmaceutical industry to tell us what to do without asking questions?

Think of how you feel when you are driving a car and have a "back seat driver" telling you how to drive. We have all been there, right? However, it becomes much less enjoyable and much more annoying when your companion starts directing you how to drive with constant commands like, "slow down" or "watch out."

This is how you should react when anyone tells you what to do! It is your life and you should be in the driver's seat. You should feel empowered to listen to your own body and follow the path that gives your body the strength to live life to the fullest! You should move your body along to the crazy dance tunes of life instead of lying lazily on your couch and then, later, lying on a hospital bed. Of course, seek advice from medical professionals. However, conduct due diligence in learning as much as you can about their recommendations. Be your own best advocate and stay in the driver's seat.

Another wise man, Adlai Stevenson, once said, "It is not the years in your life, but the life in your years that count." None of us can control how many years, days, or even seconds we have in this life. However, we can control how we spend them. Would you rather live your life gulping down the pills the pharmaceutical industry says you need, or would you rather make healthy changes now?

If you react like me, then you would rather let your body dance to the crazy tunes of life with non-stop bursts of energy. That is the way I hope you will live. You don't have to sign up for a dance class right this minute, but you can start dancing through life right now.

I want you to take control of your life and reject the idea of depending on a drug prescription to make you feel better. Do not end up like many people do, sitting on a sofa in a hospital waiting for your turn to get a drug prescription. That path only leads to a life dependent on even more prescriptions ahead. I do not want you to be against prescription drugs, but I want to empower you to look at other solutions.

You do not have to take a pill as soon as you wake up in the morning, then before your meals, after your meals and before you go to bed at night. This life, full of colorful pills, will be colorless indeed. It may seem surprising that you can expect to live your life without pills. Most people have turned a blind eye and think that bad health is their destiny. Bad health and a drug- dependent life is only your unchangeable destiny if you accept that it is and stop trying to change it.

The human brain is an extremely powerful organ. The wonder of the mind is manifested in the technology all around us. The power of human thinking has taken mankind to the moon and now gunning for Mars.

You don't have to go as far as Mars to change your destiny. You can do that right here on earth. If you are a smoker, you can start by quitting this deadly addiction. Smoking for some begins as a rebellious adventure, but it ends up in various kinds of cancers for many smokers. Quitting is one of the toughest tasks, but smokers are doing it every day. There are 1 billion smokers worldwide and 1.3 of them quit smoking every year. You can do it, too. You can quit smoking at any time and at any age. The second you do, you will begin improving your health. You can write your own destiny and be the driver of your own vehicle. You must only decide to make it happen.

I overcame my own health issues with my own determination and "no surrender attitude." I am the kind of person who is always ready and willing to go to extreme lengths to get to do what is right. I do not want to live on pills with a weak body. As a mother, I find it my responsibility to be healthy and fit so that my kids and future grandchildren can learn to live a healthy life as well. If I am taking pills throughout my day, my kids and grandchildren will expect to do just the same. Instead, I want them to live as much of a prescription-free life as possible. I want to say to them and to you, to live the life you want to live, not the life someone else has prescribed.

For me, living life on my terms means living life independent of so many prescription drugs. I make healthy living a top priority. I like to enjoy delicious foods. Most of the time, I enjoy healthy portions of the right choices of food. I take nutritional supplements continuously to support my body in wellness and health by detoxing, cleansing, repairing, restoring, and revitalizing.

In the previous chapters, I presented the devastating effects of toxins and how we are exposed to them. Drug prescriptions are toxins that can affect you in a very significant way. Making a point to stay away from prescription drugs is a simple solution to avoid toxins going directly into your body.

I am not only a wellness practitioner, but also a research scientist. Over the years I have had the opportunity to work on various drug formulations. I collected and analyzed vast amounts of data regarding these drugs. I have worked with medical, clinical, and scientific teams to create drugs to successfully treat many diseases. People used our formulas and were significantly helped and their ailments treated.

Although I was successful in helping to research and develop effective drug formulas, I was not satisfied in my heart. I was happy for the success of the companies I worked with on pharmaceuticals, but one overriding question weighed on me: "Am I really helping people cure diseases?" The answer in my mind was a big "No." I realized I was suppressing the symptoms and that they could return at any time. As the truth dawned on me, I knew I had to make changes. I knew I could not control politics, business, or the media, but I could do the right thing for others and myself.

I realized that I could help people most not by formulating and prescribing drugs, but by letting them know the causes of disease so they could assist with the prevention of disease in the first place. My "Cure the Causes" approach was born, and I now pursue it as my mission.

When I first shared my approach in "curing the causes" as an alternative or complement to pharmaceuticals, I was vehemently opposed by people in my own industry. Their opposition discouraged me for a time. Today, however, I have a clear vision to help people live their lives as they want to instead of relying on only prescription drugs. I am not anti-prescription drugs, I am pro-you!

A prescription-free life can be achieved for most people

through the process of detoxification. Once you have started an appropriate detox plan, you will begin to live your life as you want to with emotional, mental, and physical health. You will not be dependent on as many prescriptions from physicians because you will not need them anymore. Imagine a tree that has been growing in the same soil for many years. Toxic runoff and air pollution have been polluting the soil since its first days. The cure for this tree would not be to quickly cut some of the branches down, but rather take a look at the roots and the soil around it to allow the tree to flourish for many more years to come. We as humans are the same, rather than quickly cutting off some of our "branches" we need to look at what toxins are near our "roots" and cleanse them.

We can CURE THE CAUSES!

START A DETOX PLAN

Live your life as
you want to with
emotional, mental and
physical health

CHAPTER FIVE

You are the captain of your ship–welcome aboard

"Think positively and exercise daily, eat healthy, work hard, stay strong, build faith, worry less, read more, and be happy."

—*Anonymous*

BARNACLES! THIS IS not a word that we hear very often in our daily lives. This word is very important, however, in helping to explain the process of aging. For boats, barnacles are toxins that are picked up while they are at sea. As boats travel from coast to coast, barnacles attach themselves to the boat's exterior. If these barnacles are not removed in between voyages, they can eventually pose a very dangerous threat to the exterior of the boat. In fact, one of the first commands from the ship's captain upon its return from sea is for the ship to be cleaned. Captains understand the importance of keeping the exterior of the boat clean in order to preserve it and keep it safe from the harmful effects of toxic barnacles over an extended period of time.

This same concept applies to the process of aging. Many women approach the aging process with dread or even fear.

Women who are currently enjoying the essence of their youth are often the most scared about the aging process. They think that aging will bring negative changes in their appearance.

I look at the aging process as just another natural change that every human being must go through. I embrace it as a rite of passage. I know that we are each beautiful in our own way and if we continue to love ourselves, this beauty only grows as we age.

The reason the aging process is so negative for some is because of the presence of barnacles. When we go out into the world, almost every organ of our body is exposed to different kinds of barnacles, or toxins. This is especially true for your skin, the largest organ of your body. Your skin is under the greatest threat from the toxins in the environment. These barnacles can have a very negative effect if you do not take steps to constantly remove them.

Each of us has a different skin type and tone. It is important to consult with a skincare specialist or qualified dermatologist regarding the best way to care for your skin. Follow their recommendations to routinely remove barnacles from your skin just as a ship captain removes barnacles from the outside of a boat. Revitalize the outside of your body.

Boats are strong on the outside, and they are also very beautiful. The process of removing barnacles from their exterior preserves their beauty. It also keeps them safe from harmful toxins. Keeping the exterior of the boat free from barnacles also benefits the passengers within the boat because they are kept safe when the boat is in good working order.

For you as a human, the passengers inside your boat are the cells and organs inside your body. It is equally important to keep your internal organs safe from barnacles as everything inside your body is at risk of being attacked by toxins. As the captain of your body, it is your job to keep it clean both inside and out. Just as the fate of a boat depends on the intelligence and care of its captain, your body's vitality depends on you.

The health of your body will most certainly be impacted in the future by the steps you take to protect it now. If you make wise decisions regarding your health, you will be able to free yourself from all kinds of toxins and barnacles that are a threat. If you make sure that your body is cleansed of barnacles, you can avoid problems in the years to come.

It is important to understand that, although we may not be able to avoid the toxins in our environment, we can shield ourselves from the threat they pose to our bodies on a daily basis. We should keep in mind that "prevention is better than cure."

Let us again consider how a ship is protected while at sea. Ships are made of iron and it is common knowledge that iron rusts quickly when it reacts with water and air. Despite the fact that iron can rust quickly, it is still most commonly used in the construction of large ships because iron is one of the strongest metals.

How does a ship, which is made of iron that is subject to rust, keep from rusting when it is surrounded by water and air when it travels at sea? The secret is zinc, an element that shipbuilders use to protect the ship.

Shipbuilders commonly use zinc chips on the ship. To give you a little chemistry lesson, let me explain that with metals, those that have a greater reactivity are the ones that react first. Chemistry is also known as the study of chemicals and how they change. If we look at the reactivity series, which is a list that begins with the most reactive metal and ends with the least reactive metal, zinc comes before iron.

So, the reason that zinc chips are used in building ships is to protect the iron from rusting. If the iron of the ship is covered with a protective layer of zinc, then the water will react with zinc instead of iron, which completely prevents the process that causes rust.

How can you apply this same concept in protecting your body from the barnacles that are present in our atmosphere? Just as rust can destroy iron, the barnacles that are present in our atmosphere can also cause serious damage to your body. Therefore, it is necessary to use certain methods to shield both the external and internal regions of your body to protect it from the effects that toxins may have. It is essential to protect your body by supplementing with items like oregano, resveratrol, black cumin seed, turmeric, Vitamins C, E, K, D3, and zinc.

In this way, detoxification can play an important role in shielding you from the harmful effects of toxins in our atmosphere. Detoxification is like removing the barnacles from a ship, or like cleaning your house. Many people confuse the extent to which the house needs cleaning. Also, some rooms of a house, such as the kitchen, tend to need cleaning more often than others. I, personally, use different types of silicas, minerals, and zeolites to detoxify. When I make these into a formulation, I lean on my education in nutrition, science, pharmaceuticals, and nanotechnology to create personalized products so others can clean their bodies, as well!

For most of us, cleaning the kitchen is something we do daily. The kitchen is where meals are made throughout the day. If we have guests over, the kitchen might become even messier from preparing food for more people. The dishes and the sink get dirty and need to be scrubbed clean. I tend to want to procrastinate when it comes to cleaning the kitchen. I see the mess, get frustrated, and decide to delay the process of cleaning the kitchen until the next day. Unfortunately, when I do this, I find that I don't have time to clean the kitchen the next morning because I have to go to work. The kitchen stays messy. When I return from work and see the kitchen in the same disarray as the night before, frustration turns to anger because I can't cook dinner until I finally take the time to clean the kitchen.

Our bodies work much like a messy kitchen. When we delay the process of cleaning or detoxification, the process becomes even more difficult. Instead, if we take the time to "clean the kitchen" right away, we will not have to make the extra effort later. Similarly, body—detoxification should be done daily, using products that do not harm your body during the process. It doesn't matter how busy we are or how tiring it can be to take care of our bodies. The process of detoxification should be done daily. Imagine when you get up in the morning you observe that the kitchen is sparkling clean. You are able to go about your day and do what needs to be done because the kitchen is in good working order.

This can be the case with your body as well. If you take time to eat right and exercise and do everything that you have planned to take care of yourself, your body will be clean and healthy and capable of being very productive. Conversely, if you do not eat right or supplement your body with nutrition, your health can turn in a negative direction without you realizing it.

Let's circle back to the concept of barnacles on our skin. Barnacles on our skin can drastically affect the aging process. When we talk about aging, we talk about a natural process that occurs to every human being. Having traveled to over 80 countries, I've had the chance to visit Italy several times. Italy is graced by a few of the oldest buildings in the world including the Roman Coliseum, St. Peter's Basilica, and the Florence Cathedral, just to name a few. Although centuries old, these buildings still look beautiful and very pleasing to the eye. The reason is that they have been well preserved. You need to preserve your body. You have more value than any building or piece of art.

With proper care and supplements, the process of aging

can have similar results for us. It can be a blessing instead of something we fear. Barnacles on the skin are the reason the effects of aging appear the way they do. Instead, if you take care to remove the barnacles from your skin, you can experience aging gracefully. I myself have already stepped into my early fifties and I have no magic potion that keeps my skin glowing and free of wrinkles. I believe in the purity of life and do not personally use "magical" digital editing to alter my appearance in photos. The face I present to the world is the real me and not my impure digital image. I believe I am aging gracefully and that it is because of a complete detox.

You can age gracefully if you make the right choices in your life at the right time. My secret to aging is detoxification and you can adopt it right away.

Many people fear the process of aging, but it is a process that no one can ever stop. What we can do instead is age gracefully. We should welcome aging because, as we get older, we also become wiser with more experience.

Instead of being afraid of aging, we should fear the presence of barnacles on the largest organ of our bodies, which is our skin. Do not confuse the process of detoxification with a cream or potion that can be applied to the skin. The process of getting rid of barnacles requires serious commitment. Every necessary measure should be taken to remove the barnacles inside and outside of your body. You can surely win the fight if you are aggressive and meet the challenge face to face.

Like a boat, your body needs constant maintenance if you want it to work properly. The captain of a ship will never allow even a single barnacle to be left on the boat because he or she knows that even a single barnacle can have a very harmful impact.

Similarly, as the captain of your own body, you must make every effort to ensure that your body is free of barnacles. You cannot sail through your life if you are not healthy enough to sustain the daily pressures. The process of detoxification— removing barnacles—is not a one- time thing. The process can take an entire lifetime.

It may require your time and money to engage in detoxification throughout your life.

However, the best things in life require an investment both personally and financially. Many of us go on a vacation one or twice a year. We spend money on activities that we love. These are reasons that we all want to earn money in the first place. However, we should not be investing time and money on those endeavors while neglecting to spend the needed time and energy on our health.

The long-term effects that daily detox, cleaning, and restoring will have on your body are endless because as we age we become more susceptible to the negative toxins around us. As we grow older our bodies have been finding the negative all around us for longer amounts of time, and we can grow tired. By combatting this through supporting our body we will be able to have the best quality of life. Investing in your health will yield lifelong dividends. So, get your ship in order, and full steam ahead!

We can CURE THE CAUSES!

The secret to aging well
is cleaning &
detoxification

CHAPTER SIX

You will renovate a house but what will you do to improve your health

"Mainstream medicine would be way different if they focused on prevention even half as much as they focused on intervention..."

—Anonymous

HAVE YOU EVER seen a home renovation from beginning to end? Whether you have watched a home renovation television show, or even renovated a home yourself, you are probably familiar with the drastic results that can take place. Old homes can become like new again...outdated interiors can become even better than before. Homes become restored and revitalized to almost better than new!

A similar "renovation" can take place within your body. Just as we can relate cleaning a home to "cleaning" our bodies or removing "barnacles," we can take on major renovations for our health. Renovations become necessary when drastic changes are desired. If you have been living an unhealthy lifestyle for many years and have never engaged in the detoxification process, then your health may need a major renovation. The key purpose of renovating a home is the removal of the old and unused taking up space that could be enhanced with the new.

Before you decide that renovating your health sounds like it would take way too much work, or be way too expensive, let me remind you that a healthy body is worth all the time and money in the world. A healthy body is essential for you to enjoy your life to the fullest.

Today's standards for success and happiness seem to revolve around big bank accounts, fancy cars, and grand homes. The present generation has become hyper-focused on finding ways to become rich and famous. Ambition can be healthy, but it can be devastating if it is misplaced.

Being obsessed with gaining material wealth can cost you your physical, emotional, and spiritual health. Don't spend your life accumulating riches at the cost of what's more important, which is your health. If you live your life to impress others, you will never be satisfied with yourself.

You may have heard the old proverb, "health is wealth." Most of us fail to understand and apply this ancient wisdom. I want you to think about this statement and internalize it. True wealth is health. With a healthy body, you can do the things that you want to do in life that can ultimately bring you success and happiness. However, you must balance the work of life with care for yourself. If you are at your best health, you will be more effective and better focused at whatever you choose to do. I truly believe that one's ailing health is caused by the various toxins in our world. These toxins are the harmful substances that are present in our environment that can cause serious damage to you physically, emotionally, and spiritually. Thus, the detoxification process considers the physical, emotional, and spiritual components of your body.

Your body needs to be free from toxic substances in order to be healthy.

Detoxification requires a commitment, but it can be done without spending lots of money or undergoing complex procedures. Supplementing your body with essential nutrients can be a little more of an investment but can ensure that your body remains safe from all kinds of toxins.

Maintaining your health is much less costly in the long run. We should all have the same approach to our health as we do about the appearance of our homes. We are willing to invest thousands of dollars in home renovations but do not want to spend money to renovate and restore our health. Your body is like a house. You are the owner. As the owner, it is your job to make it the best it can be. A healthy body is full of positive energy that is necessary for achieving your dreams in life.

When you evaluate your "needs" versus "wants" in life, your health should be considered a top priority. Spending time and money to renovate your health is not frivolous. I'm not talking about extensive workout sessions and expensive diet plans. All it takes is a small amount of your effort and income—applied consistently—to make your body healthier. You need to make YOU a top priority!

Time is a precious asset, especially in today's fast-paced, modern world. I would never suggest that you waste time on something not worthwhile. Your health is very much worth the time and money you invest in it. What good can time and money possibly bring to us if we do not use them to take care of our health?

We humans are blessed to be the most intelligent of all creatures. Our ability to think and act intelligently makes humans superior to all living things. We cannot ignore this precious gift that nature has given us. We need to invest time and money to take care of ourselves so that we can offer the world our best selves. We have a responsibility to humanity and the earth.

I believe that humankind suffers from so many diseases today because of the collective ignorance we have of our own bodies. We have been to the moon and back, but we still do not fully understand the brilliance of the earthly vessels we inhabit. It is time to turn on energy in our own lives. We cannot help others without first helping ourselves.

We all need to ask ourselves if we are spending enough time and resources to take care of our health. In present circumstances, this question is not about winning, but about surviving. When I talk about renovating your health, I am stressing the need to protect your body from the toxins that are moving freely in our atmosphere. A house offers protection from all kinds of changes in the weather, from snowstorms to thunderstorms. Similarly, your body needs to be strong enough to withstand the storms of toxins.

The overuse of coal, oil, and gas has brought about negative changes to our planet. These changes are affecting our earth at an accelerated pace. We have chosen technology over the survival of our planet. The day we started utilizing our planet's resources without proper accountability was the day we started rushing toward our own destruction. Today, toxins are present in such great numbers that there is virtually no place left on this planet that is free of them. God has created a balance in everything. When we start affecting that balance, negative changes occur for our planet.

Detoxification is the permanent solution for protecting yourself and your children. Even greater challenges are coming our way. The world climate is changing at a drastic pace. It is our job to survive these changes and challenges. We will need strong bodies in order to do so. We have to cleanse our bodies no matter the cost.

Numerous everyday examples can help us understand the process of detoxification. For instance, cars require constant maintenance in order to be efficient and run longer. The car's engine oil must be changed from time to time in order to keep it clean and prevent breakdowns.

Our bodies are natural machines too. The maintenance they need includes detoxification on a regular basis. Your body travels daily and requires care and attention, just like a car does. Fuel and maintenance help protect the car from the harmful elements surrounding it.

Detoxification is a process that never stops. If you want to live a healthy and disease-free life, detoxification should become an essential part of your routine. It will help you look and feel your best. It is not a one-time solution. Detoxification, like renovation, will help you eliminate all kinds of toxic materials that can cause harm to your body and strengthen the areas that are weakened by attacks from toxic elements.

One of the most important functions of your body is its natural process in getting rid of harmful substances that enter it. Your liver, intestines, kidneys, lungs, and skin are all associated with the detoxification system. Together, they serve as a kind of burglar alarm that helps your body identify toxins and eliminate them. Just like a security system for your house, the security system for your body can sometimes fail. When that happens, it is important to mend the system before the intruders can inflict damage.

Detoxification is a process that aids your body's security system and makes it stronger, by eliminating toxins and avoiding substances that enable toxins to remain inside your body. Your body needs certain minerals, nutrients, and vitamins to help it eliminate the collection of toxins and other unwanted substances. It is important to use quality nutritional supplements, vitamins, and minerals to protect and support our bodies. I call it the "ABC's of Life!"

A healthy diet is the most important way to detoxify your

body. You should avoid eating processed foods and foods that contain fructose (which is found in soft drinks and sodas) that introduce toxins or interfere with the process of detoxification. Simple sugar can increase the level of toxins in our body and lead to disorders such as obesity. It is also responsible for various other problems such as chronic inflammation and stress. Overeating simple sugars can have the same effect as termites inside your house.

Food sensitivities can also contribute to toxicity in your body. Gluten, dairy, soy, and corn are foods that are most commonly associated with sensitivity. Eating these foods can make your body less reactive in eliminating toxins or keeping them from entering your body in the first place.

As I mentioned before, toxicity is not just limited to the physical toxins in our world. We can suffer from spiritual toxicity as well. Our spirits need to be detoxified regularly as well. One way to do this is through mind relaxation or meditation.

To benefit the most from spiritual detoxification through meditation, you need to eliminate as many distractions as possible. Try to meditate when you are alone and cannot be disturbed. This will help you clear away the stress and help you completely relax without worldly worries on your mind. You can also light some candles, dim or turn off the lights, and draw the curtains. You should dress comfortably for meditation. Anything that could cause a disturbance should be avoided.

Start your meditation by focusing on your breathing. Try to feel each breath as you inhale, then feel that same air as you exhale. Follow each breath from beginning to end. Slowly, you will start to flow into a relaxed state of body and mind. Then, you can choose from two paths. First, you could concentrate your energy on spiritual detoxification. Imagine any real, positive picture in your mind and move your consciousness toward that positivity. Second, you could choose to "reach out to yourself" during meditation. You can then motivate yourself to carry out spiritual detoxification while allowing your inner self to guide you through the process. It is important to not try and achieve all the results at the same time. Be patient and the results will surface themselves.

You are not completely healthy if you are not relaxed and focused in your mind. A relaxed mind and positive spirit are just as important as a clean and healthy body to keep physical and spiritual toxins at bay.

I understand that this journey can be very challenging for some, as it demands a commitment of concentration and time. Please be encouraged and know that it is not necessary to rush into or through this process. Instead, allow detoxification to slowly and gradually become part of your life. A lifestyle of detox requires years of hard work and consistency. It is important that we remain loyal to ourselves and to those around us and begin detoxifying our minds, bodies, and spirits so that we can live life with joy and peace. It is important to surround ourselves with other people dedicated to this mission.

We can CURE THE CAUSES!

Health is wealth

CHAPTER SEVEN

Living with environmental toxins

"You can renovate your health in the world you live in."

—*Dr. Christina Rahm*

IN TODAY'S MODERN world, we are surrounded by a host of toxins. Many of these toxins are byproducts of industry, which became the main source of income for many countries at the start of the industrial revolution in Europe a few centuries ago. These age-old toxins are constantly attacking our body. In order to take on this daily battle of fighting these toxins, we need to better understand what is going on in the environment around us.

Industrialists have not owned up to the role industry has played in causing serious damage to the environment. Furthermore, humanity has allowed the industry to continue to prosper and release toxins into the environment. Decades have gone by as companies have depleted many of the planet's major resources while continuously releasing toxins into the environment.

The level of toxicity within our environment today is higher than ever and we are faced with diseases that were once unheard of. Nature must have known that humans would someday be destructive and harmful to the planet. Therefore, our bodies are born with a natural support system that acts as a protective shield against harmful toxins. However, our natural defenses are no longer enough to defend us against the strength of the toxins surrounding us. Furthermore, our lifestyles have caused the natural cleaning systems of our bodies to suffer greatly.

Each of us is within the grasp of harmful substances. Technological advancement has brought about easy living and lack of physicality, which is making us unhealthy. Industrial and technological advancement is destroying us! We are standing on the edge of the limit that our bodies can take. We must not push this limit any further. Instead, we must muster the strength and resources we need to counter these dangerous elements and win the battle of survival.

The first step is to support your body's natural cleansing system. There are simple habits that can bring about very positive changes. I recommend drinking plenty of water, at least twelve, eight-ounce glasses per day combined with additional support from natural detox products. When possible, you should also keep an organic diet at a minimum and avoid using plastic or consuming foods that have been wrapped in plastic food packaging.

Even seemingly small habits can bring about very positive changes. Gradually, you will become a healthier person with a new sense of motivation. You must also supplement and restore your body daily with vitamins and minerals. As the toxins in our environment have increased, the presence of essential vitamins and minerals has diminished. Our environment can no longer provide enough minerals and vitamins for our bodies. Thus, it is our responsibility to ensure we give our bodies the elements they need.

Few people understand the vital role that vitamins and

minerals play in human health. It is your responsibility to acquire proper knowledge in relation to the vitamins and minerals your body needs.

Vitamins and minerals also have a role in cleansing your body. Cleaning your body is a responsibility that falls upon you and you alone. You cannot expect your friends, parents, or spouse to carry out this task for you. There are several natural methods that can be used to detoxify your body. This process is termed "natural detox." Products that have essentials like magnesium, silicas, Vitamins A, B, C, etc., zinc, niacin olive leaf, oregano, resveratrol, etc. can assist your body by supporting wellness daily.

You may think natural detox will involve very difficult procedures and methods, but that is not the case at all. Natural detox is a very simple and easy way to clean yourself from the harmful toxins that might be present within your body. Our bodies have a very amazing natural resistance to toxins, but as the toxins in our environment have grown in strength, our resistance to them has diminished. Natural detox supports your body's internal purification system. I have formulated products with Root Wellness and ABC's For Life to assist the body in doing just this! I wanted everyone to have access to products that can simply and gently cleanse their bodies and improve their lives! I continue to hope these products or similar, will assist others in having a healthier, happier life.

As I have stated previously in this book when it comes to your body, you are in control; you are the mayor. You are the only one who can make decisions regarding your body. No one else can do this for you. Do not allow other people or circumstances to dictate your own health. Support your body's natural systems to help improve them and make them more efficient.

Each of us has responsibility for the care of our own bodies. However, we must all take responsibility for the environment. We must make sure that our environment is as clean as it should be. We cannot expect a positive outcome for human health if we continue to surround ourselves with toxins for future generations.

There are many methods that can be used to create a healthy environment for you and your family. The practice of keeping your environment clean should be done on a regular basis. You cannot expect a clean home every day if you only clean it once a month. The process of cleaning your body and the environment requires consistency in order to produce optimal results. The products I formulated with Root Wellness are purposely gentle enough for daily use for most people. These are not the only products you can use. Choose products from companies whose ingredient sourcing, scientists, and management you can trust. Choosing the right company for your nutritional supplements is as important as choosing the builder of your home. Because your body is your permanent home!

I cannot overstate the immediate threat that our current environment poses to all of us, especially children. Therefore, conducting environmental detox is imperative. An efficient environmental detox includes correcting diet, addressing environmental toxins, removing bad bacteria, and repopulating your body with healthy minerals and vitamins to help all vital organs work efficiently and properly.

To ensure the best results, you should review your plans for an environmental detoxification with a professional medical practitioner and an environmentalist. They can help you address any individual concerns that may arise and help ensure that you are completing the steps of detoxification in the correct order. The above method of conducting an environmental detox can result in a great improvement in your entire well-being! People who suffer from diseases caused by the toxins present in our surroundings often find that their symptoms are completely resolved after undergoing environmental detox.

It must be understood, however, that professional guidance is essential. The process of detoxification does not need to be unpleasant. If you are properly supervised under the care of a professional, you should not experience the discomfort of any sort.

In order to live a life that is completely free of toxins, we must adopt the process of detoxification and implement it for ourselves and for the environment. If we put this into practice, future generations could be kept safe from the various diseases that are becoming increasingly common today. Detoxification, combined with a wellness plan, can protect human health as well as the health of the environment.

Today, I witness many people living an unhealthy lifestyle. They are unaware of how far they are along the road of destruction. The importance of a healthy lifestyle has been minimized and almost forgotten in modern culture. Again, I want to state that each of us is the "mayor" of our own body. We must protect it against dangerous toxins. This should be your priority.

If you are blessed to be a parent, you have an amazing opportunity to instill healthy habits in your children. Many children today are becoming less active outside and more involved in indoor activities involving electronics. The importance and necessity of physical activity is being overlooked. Many factors contribute to this, such as the busy schedule that most families keep. The result, however, is that childhood obesity is on the rise.

For children to live a healthy, toxin-free life, it is important to introduce them to the importance of living an active lifestyle. As their parent, you can help them understand the responsibility they have toward their own body. You can teach them that their own natural cleansing system needs their help. You can help them develop a lifestyle of healthy living that can help them live a long, healthy life. We all need to realize the threat toxins pose to our kids. Now is the time to act!

Throughout this book, I have been trying to broaden your understanding of how your body works using everyday examples. As I discussed in the previous chapter, I see our bodies as houses that are strong, yet require constant care in order to be able to withstand the dangerous storms of life. Just like a house, the human body is as good as its owner keeps it. We all know what happens to a home if it not cleaned and maintained. The same can happen with the human body. Without consistent care and cleansing, the body cannot stay strong.

When it comes to renovating a house, some areas may need more extensive renovation and restoration than others. This again applies to the human body. Some areas of health may need minor tweaks, while others need drastic improvement. From the outside, a home can look beautiful but have an interior that is in disrepair. Similarly, a person can look happy and healthy on the outside but have an unhealthy lifestyle that is taking its toll on their overall life.

You must be honest with yourself about the lifestyle changes you need to make. No one else can really do this for you. It is easy to hide unhealthy habits from family and friends for a while. Eventually, poor lifestyle choices will take their toll.

Own up to your bad habits before it is too late. Don't try to deliberately ignore areas of your health that need attention.

Face them and seek the help you need. Many other people in your life can be affected by your unhealthy living. Each of us must take responsibility for our own body and do what needs to be done to be as healthy as possible.

We can CURE THE CAUSES!

Own up to bad habits
Live a healthy life

CHAPTER EIGHT

Your workplace is no exception for detox

"We do not inherit the earth from our ancestors, we borrow it from our children."

—*Native American Proverb*

WE SPEND MUCH of our daily lives working. How we feel while we are at our place of work can greatly impact our wellbeing. The workplace can either be a place that inspires us and lifts us up, or it can be a place of dread that drags us down.

The way your workplace makes you feel is a good indicator of whether it is a toxic environment. Many factors can contribute to workplace toxicity. There are two types of toxicity that affect the workplace, emotional and physical. Emotional toxicity relates to human nature and interpersonal behavior. Physical toxicity concerns physical hazards in the workplace that can be harmful to human health.

Let's first discuss physical toxicity in the workplace. Employers have a great responsibility to create a safe workplace. Some employees may tolerate an unsafe work environment in order to maintain a job that provides for their families.

These employees can be the most vulnerable to a physically toxic work environment. As we have learned in the previous chapters, physical toxicity is extremely harmful to human health. Nothing has brought this into the open more than the SARS2 pandemic and other viruses. It is important to protect your bodies at home, at work, and in your community.

Potentially toxic substances in the workplace that are documented to have caused the injury in certain situations include paint, lead, pesticides, asbestos, solvents, benzene, mercury, silica, beryllium, vinyl, chloride, cadmium, acids, plastics in production, exhaust or welding materials, just to name a few. Workers must avoid exposure to such substances. If they must come into contact with harmful substances, viruses, bacteria, etc. they need to have gloves, eye protection, helmets, or even bodysuits if needed. Workspaces must be properly ventilated. Medical attention must be sought immediately upon exposure to harmful substances or viruses.

Employees should be empowered to utilize any safety equipment available. Workplace culture should encourage employees to follow safety precautions. Time must be allowed to put on proper attire and safety equipment. Every person in the company should be educated about the risks of working in or around potentially harmful substances and take a pro-active stance to avoid injury. Everyone should be encouraged to take charge of their own personal wellness.

Hazardous jobs, such as coal mining and mineral extraction, can be the most concerning. Jobs in the construction industry can pose dangers to employees as well. Companies that employ workers in such fields must take even more safety measures and provide training and adequate safety equipment. Precautions must be taken to prevent workers from breathing in toxic fumes that can lead to lung and throat infections and cancers.

Now let's look at emotional toxicity in the workplace. Emotional toxicity stems from negative interpersonal interactions. Poor culture can foster negative feelings among employees. If people do not feel emotionally safe at work, their entire psyche is affected. Employers have a great responsibility to create a place of work where people feel celebrated and supported. There is no room for discrimination. In fact, inequality in the workplace is highly toxic.

When people are discriminated against, their health and well-being are impacted. No one should have to deal with the emotional stress that comes with discrimination in the workplace. Furthermore, the toxic stress a person feels during the workday can follow them home and impact every aspect of their life. If discrimination affects their pay, they will feel disappointment and shame every time they face the bills they need to pay.

In today's economy, companies can make tremendous amounts of money. However, profit should never come at the expense of those who are the backbone of the economy. When people are not valued, it truly affects everyone. Alternatively, when people do feel valued, they contribute the best of themselves to the organizations they are a part of. Human ingenuity is beyond measure.

Inequality can be bold or subtle. It can rear its ugly head in obvious ways that cause people to be treated differently because of race, gender, or social standing. Inequality can also be a more subtle, underlying tone in the workplace that is harder to pinpoint. It can be part of the culture that gives preference to management levels and tenure. Whether bold or subtle, inequality in the workplace is negative and highly toxic. Sometimes, toxicity can be traced back through many years of company history. It is important to take a stance against this toxicity.

If you are in a position of leadership in your company, be on the lookout for negativity. If a team member seems shrouded in the negativity that is affecting both the team and the individual themselves, talk to that person. Try to understand what they are going through. Often, people are struggling with personal situations that overflow and project into their work. They may need help seeking solutions for positive change. While you are helping that person, be sure to document every conversation and try to limit negative interactions. Never discuss one team member with another team member, but welcome candid conversations and feedback if another team member is helping to bring your attention to a negative situation. Try to keep the negativity from overwhelming the positive change that can take place.

No matter your role in the company, if your place of work is toxic, you must do everything you can to detoxify it. If you are in a position of influence in the company, begin to speak up as an agent for change. Be on the lookout for the subtle signs of discrimination and equality. Advocate for those who are not able to advocate for themselves. Remember, a toxic work environment negatively affects everyone involved. It is worth fighting for change.

If your work environment is toxic, but you find that you cannot effectively change it, I strongly advise you to seek another solution. Do everything you can to find a place of employment that is positive for you. Even if you accept less pay in exchange for a healthy work environment, you will be making the best choice for your long-term future. Stress and negativity are highly toxic and can be detrimental to your health and well-being.

I hope as you are reading this book your eyes are being opened to the world around you and the effects it has on you personally. We are all connected. What happens in our homes, places of work and communities affects us all in either positive or negative ways. When you become aware of things that affect you negatively, you can find ways to change. I hope you will find the courage to do this as you continue reading. Change can be difficult, but it is worth it.

On the bright side, employers are becoming more conscious of their employees' well-being. They are working to create team-focused environments that celebrate the contributions of all employees. They are initiating "no tolerance" policies when it comes to discrimination. Some executives have even issued "no door" or "open door" policies, rejecting the "corner office syndrome."

Promoting health and wellness in the workplace is becoming more common. Employers are recognizing the benefits of making the health of their employees a priority. Wellness initiatives are a win-win for employers and employees. Research has shown when employee wellness is prioritized, absenteeism decreases, while employee satisfaction and productivity increase. The health of the workplace itself should be as much a concern as the health of individual employees. Everyone can work together to detoxify the workplace.

There must be a micro and macro approach to environmental detox in the workplace.

Creating a healthier workplace is good for the individuals who work for a company and good on a larger scale for the environment and human health. Companies cannot get so caught up in being politically correct and environmentally conscious that they neglect the health of the very people who make up their organization. The health and wellbeing of employees should be as important as the environmental impact of a company.

Every challenge in life is an opportunity to succeed. You can protect your workplace from toxins born of human behavior and those that are part of the physical environment. We can cure the cause of workplace toxicity by being introspective, retrospective and proactive. We can each do what we can to do take charge of the elements and situations we have influence over. We can work together toward positive change to make the workplace a safer and healthier place.

We can CURE THE CAUSES!

PROMOTE HEALTH & WELLNESS IN THE WORKPLACE

CHAPTER NINE
Anti-aging and skincare

"It's not how old you are, it's how you are old."

—*Jules Renard*

A NTI-AGING IS A state of mind, and body. As a society, we tend to focus on the change in physicality that occurs with aging. Yet, we fail to notice the benefits of aging such as the wisdom and maturity that can only be gained through years of living. If we correct our state of mind to see getting older as the blessing that it is, our countenance will project ageless grace. We can embody the adage and "grow old gracefully."

Women are especially vulnerable to negative feelings about aging. They equate aging with loss of beauty and, therefore, value. This is a tragic misconception at the core of our culture. The value of a woman is not based on physical beauty. Each woman has immeasurable value.

Women who impart this knowledge to their innermost being find immunity from the fickle opinions the world may have about their age.

For me, the changes time brings are what make life more fun and interesting. While being in your twenties can be fun and exciting, our later years are full of riches a twenty-something cannot even fully understand. In my experience, when I ask someone to recount their twenties, they generally tell me about all the risks they took, the poor decisions they made, and the things they wished they would have known back then!

As we work on our state of mind to help us age gracefully, we can also do things to complement the aging process physically. Just as a house needs to be maintained, so does your skin. There are minor practices that will keep your house clean and strong. The same is true for your skin.

I introduced the concept of "barnacles" earlier in this book. Our skin's surface has barnacles that must be removed regularly in order to prevent their ill effects. The skin is the largest organ of your body. It is subject to having barnacles on the outside and on the inside. In order to protect the skin, barnacles must be removed through the process of detoxification. Just as the issues of a city are not cosmetic, the effects of toxicity are more than skin deep. They are systemic. Detoxification is a process that applies to your entire body. You cannot be free of toxins unless your body is completely cleaned. You must keep yourself and your environment as clean as possible. Steps to do this must be taken on a regular basis; this is a 365-day-a-year process.

You should also take steps to supplement your body. By supplementing, I do not mean that you can just take a few pills on the weekend and consider the job done. Detoxification and supplementation must be done regularly if you wish to achieve a positive result. They must also be done by using the right products. Many nutritional companies cut corners by choosing the cheapest ingredients. Make sure to know the companies that produce the products you use.

In their quest to combat aging, many people—especially women because of their vulnerability on this subject—tend to purchase skin care products that promise fast results.

Manufacturers of such products make those claims in order to increase profits; they have little to do with actual skincare. They may produce results quickly, but they will only be temporary, artificial changes that will fade away just as quickly as they came. I advise staying away from such products as they can have a negative impact on your body and your emotional state. True skincare will bring about lasting results. The results will take time and consistency to achieve, but they will be worth it. It is important to focus on supplementing your body to shield it from the toxins that can have very harmful effects instead of looking for shortcuts. To have the greatest impact on your outsides, you must detoxify on the inside.

By supplementing your body with good things, you can become a person who is full of energy and has a positive glow. A big mistake many people make is believing in the advertising of a product and not the science behind it. This can lead to skin, and health, problems because you are not using products that are supporting your cells. Always take a closer look at the products that you are putting on your body because chances are it could have some harmful ingredients. You cannot avoid aging but taking care of your skin with nutrient-dense products will help you to be healthy and feel beautiful.

To further understand skincare as it relates to aging, it is important to understand how the body works. In today's world, dangerous toxins surround us and cause serious damage to our organs. Since our skin is the largest organ of the body, it suffers the most. We need to revitalize your skin!

When you travel, you must be especially aware of the exposure to different toxins that can have very harmful effects. You can "wash" your body through anti-toxin supplements. After you return from a journey, it is necessary to undergo a "power-wash" to remove the effects of the additional exposure to toxins.

The dangers of pollution can be seen in the various diseases that are present in our world that were unheard of just a few decades ago. Many of these diseases affect the skin and are the result of increased exposure to toxins and heavy metals in our atmosphere. Just as a soldier needs armor before stepping into battle, your body needs armor against the harmful effects of the environment.

The human body needs supplements in order to defend against toxins in the environment. It is important to consult a professional regarding this. Before you use anything on your skin, you must be sure that the solution does not end up being more of a problem. Again, keep in mind that consistency is the key. Every product, supplement, or remedy requires proper time in order to detoxify. Since the toxins in our environment are much stronger than before, we should allow more time for supplements and detoxification to do their work.

As the title of this book suggests, I place my focus on the causes of the health problems we have. I truly believe that we must cure by correcting the causes of disease. If we eliminate the things that are causing negative changes to our bodies, we can live longer and become who we are truly meant to be. This is the very basis behind the powerful-yet-gentle detox supplements I formulated for Root Wellness, and this will also be the case for the products coming from a new line I have founded. ABC's For Life will help you detox through the apparel you wear, your beauty routine, and even decrease the toxicity of the beverages you drink.

No matter what we do, as we age, our bodies will change. How we perceive those changes will have more of an effect than the changes themselves. Your body reflects your personality. If you are a positive person who considers life to be a blessing and does everything to make it healthier and more exciting, your body and outward appearance will indeed reflect it.

I want to emphasize the importance of skincare as it applies to overall health. The skin is the vanguard of the rest of the body. It is our security system. Nature has provided this vital shield to protect our bodies. It falls upon us to make sure that we take care of it and keep it free of toxins that can cause damage to it. A person who has a negative attitude toward health and aging will invite emotional and spiritual toxins into their life that will compound the effects of physical toxins. Overall, enjoy the journey to health. Do not be in a hurry to run toward a specific goal. The ride is always more exciting than the destination.

We can CURE THE CAUSES!

Taking care of your skin
will help you to be healthy
and feel beautiful

CHAPTER TEN

Protect your children and keep them healthy for life

"History will judge us by the difference we make in the everyday lives of children."

—*Nelson Mandela*

THE FUTURE OF humanity is our children. As a mother of four, I can tell you that being a mom is one of the most incredible experiences on earth. I love all my children with all my being. I would do anything for them. When I see expecting mothers or newborn babies, I can hardly contain my excitement. The joy that children bring to our world is immeasurable.

The blessings of children come with responsibility for all of us. We must take steps to secure the health and environment for our present and future generations.

Our environment is contaminated with toxic substances. The moment a baby is born, he or she is exposed to these harmful toxins. As an infant, a baby is most vulnerable to the effects of toxins. They grow stronger as they get older, but the toxins are still all around them. Even the food they eat is contaminated with toxins and pollutants. These toxins affect children throughout their lives. Research shows that many childhood conditions are increasing at an alarming rate as a result of the prevalence of toxins in our world.

To combat the harmful effects of toxins, we must train our kids to win this battle. Just like in movies that portray a young child that trains to become a warrior and grows up to win an epic battle, we must help our kids learn to win against toxins. The weapons will be knowledge about detoxification and healthy lifestyle choices.

Contortion artists can flex and bend their bodies into seemingly impossible poses. Many of them began training at a very young age because we are much more flexible as children than as adults. Skills are much more profound if taught from an early age. We can train our kids to eat cleanly at an early age so that they do not gather toxins in their bodies. We can help them prevent disease and lead healthy, active lives.

If you are a parent, I hope you will also consider the lifestyle choices that you make. Children learn much more from what we do than from what we say. For instance, you may teach your children that soft drinks are bad for their health. Then, they see that you drink soft drinks every day. Your words will seem empty to them.

Energy tends to trickle down, whether it is good or bad. Good energy will have a positive impact on your kids and everyone around you. Bad energy will make situations right under your own nose even worse. If you keep your mind positive, you will be able to transfer bursts of positive energy to others, including your kids. It might seem like a far-fetched idea, but we can all see a positive change if we project positive energy. Your kids will take this even further into their own lives as they grow up. This positive energy will help them zero in on life!

I have worked with children in counseling and studied neuropsychology. I can tell you that the lessons taught in childhood—good or bad—are extremely difficult to overcome. What you teach your children when they are young will shape their habits as they grow into adults.

Clean eating is one of the most important habits you can establish in your children. Good eating habits can positively impact your child's health throughout their life. You can also teach them practices that reduce their exposure to toxins. For example, encourage your children to remove their shoes before walking into the house. Explain that shoes can carry harmful germs, so it is best to leave them at the door. You can even place a basket or mat by the door as a reminder.

Do everything you can to minimize the exposure to toxic substances in your home. When you buy cleaning or personal care products—especially those for children—read the labels and avoid products with potentially hazardous chemicals.

You can also help your children learn to eat detoxifying foods that can help their body to cleanse itself. Eating detoxifying food is one of the best ways to detoxify your body. Naturally detoxifying foods include herbs and nutrients that can fortify the body against toxins.

Probiotics are very important to overall health. Your digestive system has good and bad bacteria. The healthy bacteria that line the gut help to break down toxins in the GI tract and liver. The bad bacteria decrease your body's capability to cleanse and remove toxins. The major sources of probiotics include supplements and foods such as yogurt. Including yogurt in your child's diet can also aid in digestion and regeneration.

Prebiotics are just as vital as probiotics. They help the healthy bacteria grow. Foods that are rich in prebiotics include artichokes, onions, leeks, and asparagus. There are also wonderful supplements I often recommend to my clients that contain prebiotics and probiotics. Further, if you can find the right products made with colostrum, clinoptilolite, silica, and collagen.

Fiber binds toxins and takes them out of the body through the digestive tract. Foods that are rich in fiber include fruits such as bananas, mangoes, oranges, apples, and vegetables such as peas, broccoli, and Brussels sprouts. Beans, legumes, and nuts are also good sources of fiber.

Some vegetables contain isothiocyanates that support the body's resistance to toxins. These are brassica vegetables such as broccoli, cabbage, cauliflower, collards, kale, and bok choy.

Ellagic Acid is a very strong antioxidant that enhances the liver's detoxifying enzymes.

Ellagic acid is found in pomegranate juice, cranberries, purple grapes, pecans, walnuts, and most kinds of berries.

Other detoxifying foods include turmeric, garlic, and B vitamins. When you focus on including these foods in your own diet and encourage your kids to eat them as well, you will be building healthy habits that will benefit them for life and help them be strong against the effects of toxins.

We can CURE THE CAUSES!

The weapons against toxins are knowledge about detoxification and healthy lifestyle choices

CHAPTER ELEVEN
Dance to detox

"Physical fitness is not only one of the most important keys to a healthy body, it is the basis of dynamic and creative intellectual activity"

—*John F. Kennedy*

EXERCISE HAS PHYSICAL as well as intellectual perks to offer. Exercise can also help you eliminate toxins from your body. The benefits of exercise are not realized as often as they should be in the sedentary world we live in today. Technology and activities such as social media have "chained us" to our seats and devices.

Physical exercise in general is one of the best ways to deal with stress and other emotional and mental toxins. Yet, it is often one of the most under-explored options in dealing with these factors. Exercise clears the mind and allows you to feel more in control of your well-being. You will also see your sleep improve, which will benefit your state of mind. Amazing things happen when your mind is clear and positive.

Not only can exercise be beneficial for your health in many ways, but it can also be fun if you have the right approach! I have developed an exercise plan that I call "Dance to Detox."

These exercises target toxins that gather in our bodies that can cause physical, mental, and emotional damage. If you think of exercise in the same way that you think of dancing, you will look forward to it and embrace it.

If you make these workouts a regular part of your daily routine, you will experience the greatest benefits of the reduction of toxins. Your workouts don't have to be long workouts. Even 15 to 20 minutes a day can jump-start your metabolism and kick your body into high alert! As you rid your body of toxins through exercise, you will feel healthier and more active than you ever have.

The first exercise I recommend is a "Restorative Yoga/Pilates workout." This type of exercise helps to stretch your muscles. Stretching can reduce pressure and stress, which can give you more mental peace and clarity. A yoga/Pilates workout is a great way to practice self-care as it provides relaxation as well as physical exercise.

You can do this exercise at any time. If you are feeling a bit run down mentally, physically, or emotionally, this restorative workout can help you combat those feelings. It is extremely beneficial for your body. The stretches and light movement help improve circulation without putting too much stress on your body. This is also a good workout to do if you do not want to engage in a more intense, complex training workout, but would still like to benefit from the physical exercise and relaxation. You will feel your mood lift and your mind relax as you go through the movements.

Another exercise I recommend is "Rebounding." Rebounding is a low-impact exercise that is usually performed on a device that is like a mini-trampoline. Rebounding is extremely beneficial for your health as it supports the proper functioning of all internal organs. It is also great fun!

When you jump on a rebounder, you are working against

the gravitational pull. When you land, the cells in your body contract, which helps them rid of waste. Increased circulation during this type of exercise provides your cells with oxygen and nutrients from your bloodstream.

The motion of a Rebounding workout also activates the lymphatic system. Your lymphatic system is a network of tissues and organs that help rid the body of toxins. The lymphatic system also transports lymph, a fluid that contains infection-fighting white blood cells throughout the body. Substances that are bad for your body, such as heavy metals and other toxins, get thrown out through the lymphatic system. Blood is pumped through your body by your heart. The lymphatic system does not have an organ that provides this function. It requires active movement to start the flow of lymph. Human beings have more lymph in their bodies than blood.

In addition to exercise, meditation is another way of relaxing your mind and detoxifying your body. There are a few simple steps to follow. First, find a quiet, peaceful place and sit down. You can sit on a chair or bench or even the floor. If you prefer to sit on the floor, you might want to have a cushion to sit on so that you will be comfortable. Begin by concentrating on the lower region of your body, your legs, feet, and bottom. If you are seated on the floor, it might be beneficial to cross your legs. Make sure your knees are at the same level as or below your hips, or else you will become uncomfortable. If you are seated on a chair, have your feet flat on the floor. Slowly move your focus to the upper region of your body. Try leaning over a bit at first to allow yourself to calm down. Then, lift your body up. Keep your spinal cord straight, but not so straight that you feel stiff. Just let your spine blend into its natural shape. If you have back issues, move into whatever upright position is most comfortable for you.

Move your focus from your back and spine to your arms and hands. The upper part of your arms should be parallel to your torso. Allow your hands to fall and rest naturally. Be mindful that you do not hunch over.

Relax your chin and allow your eyes to lower. Think of

assuming a humble posture. You can allow your eyes to close. Feel them relax as they do so much work and indeed require rest.

Meditation is a time to relax your eyes.

Focus on your mind and body coming together. Feel the contact points of your body. Feel your feet touch the floor, or your legs against the cushion.

Begin to pay special attention to your breath. Notice your breath going out and coming in. You may notice all kinds of thoughts that are entering your mind. Just let them move and be there. Bring your mind back to being present in your body. If there are thoughts that are troubling you, set them aside and know that you can come back to them.

Keep this practice going for several minutes, or even longer if you can. When you are ready, take one more deep breath in and let it out completely. Then, open your eyes. Notice that you feel refreshed from taking a mental break during your day.

The combination of meditation and exercise will have you dancing your way to detox in no time. You will feel more relaxed and vigorous than ever before. Making these practices a part of your daily routine will help your body get rid of the toxins that can weigh you down physically, mentally, and emotionally.

We can CURE THE CAUSES!

Meditate Exercise

Dance your way to detox

CHAPTER TWELVE

Let's clean your diet

"You are what you eat"

—*Anthelme Brillat-Savarin*

FOOD IS THE source of energy for our bodies. It is also one of the biggest sources of toxins.

When we consume prepackaged highly processed, or inorganic foods, we are exposing ourselves to toxins. Our bodies have a limited capability to remove the toxic trash that we consume. Food is the fuel we depend on. Would you put contaminated fuel in your car? Of course not, however, we put food that is contaminated with toxins into our bodies every day.

Part of the problem is that we do not understand the levels of toxins that can be found in food. Most of us make unhealthy food choices because we do not fully realize the potential risk to our health. What we depend on as a source of energy is a carrier of toxic chemicals and pollutants.

When we combine this with the environmental toxins our bodies are subject to, it is a double whammy. Systemic toxicity creates a negative feedback loop of more desire to consume more toxic foods.

To turn this situation around, we must admit that we have bad eating habits and acknowledge how they affect our health. Processed junk foods are really feeding the profitability of their manufacturers. We may be tempted by these foods and the advertisements suggesting them, but we still have a choice to eat them or not. You can be empowered with the right information that will help you stay strong and not be fooled by the lure of junk food. Instead of trying to make or force dietary changes, the detoxification of your body creates desires for healthier foods.

Making good choices can enable us to live a good life. Our diet is a major choice that we can make for better or for worse. Make the decision to eat cleanly and detoxify your body and you will have more energy and feel healthier. As the Chairman of the Board of the International Science Nutrition Society, I hope to enable others to make scientifically informed decisions about the way they nourish their bodies.

I want to point out that a detox diet is not about starving or eliminating food altogether for any amount of time. Your body has nutritional requirements that must be met. I strongly discourage so-called "detox diets" that do not allow you to eat solid foods. Your body is meant to receive real food. Depriving your body of food will cause a nutritional deficit.

I recommend a balanced approach. This is the "complete package" that does not require you to compromise on taste or nutrition. It is not the food itself that causes problems, but rather how the food is grown, processed, stored, and cooked. Technology has greatly influenced the food industry and I do not believe this influence to be all for the good. We should be able to eat all the different foods that nature has provided for us.

I recently took a trip where I had the chance to eat at a restaurant that was right off a fishing dock. It was fun to eat fish that had been caught fresh. However, I have a keen eye for observation. I noticed that although the fish was fresh and tasty, the water it had been swimming in was very polluted. What could have been a very healthy meal was not healthy at all because of environmental pollution.

This is an example that illustrates my point about the food we eat. Nature has provided us with many wonderful, healthy foods. What we are doing to the environment is making our food toxic. On top of that, processing food adds further toxins while taking away nutrients.

We are trapped in a vicious cycle. As we are developing more technology, we are diminishing our quality of life. Food is best served as nature intended it to be, not as science has made it.

One of the ways in which technology affects our food is through genetic engineering and bioengineering. Genetically Modified Organisms (GMOs) are living organisms whose genetic structure has been manipulated in a lab using genetic engineering. Genetic changes are applied to make crops produce more and be able to endure applications of pesticides. The scientific community is not in agreement about the safety of GMOs as food. In 2015, 300 scientists, physicians, and scholars participated in a discussion on the safety of GMOs held by the Environmental Sciences Europe. They unanimously denied the claim that GMOs are safe, leaving the discussion open for further research. Still, there are mixed reviews about GMOs being 100% safe. I see that positive feedback is biased as it comes from the biotechnology companies and their associates. However, as a nanotechnologist, I can see both sides. There can be good GMOs and bad GMOs. The problem is that most GMO technology that is good generally focuses on increasing crop yields and reducing chemical pesticides. This has been helpful for items like cotton. However, as it pertains to human consumption it is widely agreed by scientists that most GMOs can be detrimental to our health and wellness.

Another issue with GMO foods is labeling. Their labeling is not a worldwide practice yet. So far, there are 64 countries that enforce the labeling of GMO foods. All European Union countries, Russia, Australia, and Japan practice it. In Canada and the USA, it has not become an enforced practice yet. However, the U.S. Secretary of Agriculture, Sonny Perdue, announced the National Bioengineered Food Disclosure Standard (NBFDS) passed by Congress in July of 2016. Under this law, USDA will enforce the mandatory standard practice of labeling GMO foods by 2022. The law will apply to all manufacturers, importers, and retailers to label GMO foods properly.

I am a part of the bioscience-engineering and nanotechnology program at Harvard University, but I do not want to hide the truth. Personally, I am in favor that this can positively impact world hunger. However, I am not in favor of GMO foods if there is a choice. I am a proponent of organic methods for growing crops. A diet aimed at detoxification cannot contain GMO foods. Recipes that I will share in this book are recommended with organic ingredients.

Another aspect of concern is the use of pesticides because they contain toxic substances. Pests threaten many crops. To grow crops, farmers spray chemical formulas, known as pesticides, on the plants to deter pests. As crops are watered, chemicals reach the soil and are absorbed. Then, as plants absorb moisture and nutrients from the soil, they absorb the harmful chemicals as well. In this way, dangerous chemicals become part of the crops.

Crops that have been treated with harmful pesticides retain those chemicals after harvest.

When animals and humans eat the produce, they consume the toxins as well. Humans are further exposed when they eat the meat of animals that have fed on contaminated grass.

I use the term "organic" when talking about healthy foods. In a detox diet plan, the term "organic" refers to crops grown without the use of synthetic pesticides, fertilizers, genetically modified organisms, or ionizing radiation. To be part of a healthy detox diet, animal food products such as eggs, dairy, poultry, and beef should come from animals not injected with antibiotics or growth hormones.

The healthiest foods should be grown with no exposure to chemicals in any form. Organic farming methods not only produce healthier food, but they also support the environment by enhancing the overall health of the soil. There are also many organic, non-GMO, vegan supplements that can support your health and wellness. Choose these instead of choosing candy bars or junk food!

It is important to be aware of the regulations that apply to labeling foods as organic. Let's begin with a brief overview of the process a farm must undergo to be considered an organic farm. To prepare an organic farm, a farmer spends two years converting the land to organic land. Crops grown within the first year of this process are not organic. Crops grown during the second year are labeled "In Conversion." Produce grown the third year is labeled 100% organic.

In the USA, the National Organic Program (NOP) regulates organic food. Organic farmers need certification by a government-approved certifier before they can label their products as organic. The land is inspected before the certification is issued.

Not all organic labels are equal! Consumers should beware of purchasing foods labeled organic without understanding all of the facts. The United States Department of Agriculture

(USDA) has divided organic food labeling into four categories. Produce that is 100% organic will bear the USDA Organic seal. This label signifies pure organic contents. These products are the best choice for your diet and the category I most highly recommend.

The second category of organic food labels indicate that there are 95–99% organic ingredients in the product. The other added ingredients have also been approved by the NOP for use. You may also see the USDA Organic seal. This category is the second-best option.

The third category of organic food labels indicates the product has been "made with organic ingredients." This means that the percentage of organic ingredients is between 70% and 94%. You may not see the USDA Organic seal on the label; however, the manufacturer may include up to three organic ingredients on the front. Comparatively, this is still a better option than inorganic foods.

The fourth category is for products that contain less than 70% organic ingredients listed on the side panel of the product packaging. The manufacturer cannot use the USDA Organic seal on the product packaging or make any claims pertaining to organic ingredients. I do not recommend foods labeled in this category.

Organic foods can sometimes be priced a little higher than inorganic foods. Reasons for this include lack of federal subsidies and increased labor needed to grow foods organically. Organic farms are also often smaller than conventional farms. Since there are multiple food categories, you can find one that is affordable to you. It is important to keep in mind that your food choices pertain to your health. You should be kind to yourself and make the best choice that you can.

Global sales of organic foods are increasing. In 2017, the global sales of organic foods amounted to $97 billion in comparison of $90 billion in 2016. The biggest markets for organic food demand include the USA, Germany, and France. If we all turn to organic foods, it can be expected that the prices will come to a moderate level.

Another concern in food source pertains to "hydrogenated fats and oils." That may sound like a fancy and delicious term, but it is bad for your health. The fats and oils that are used to process food are commonly known as "trans fats." Trans fats are found in many food products such as baked items, snacks, fried foods, refrigerated dough, cream, and many kinds of margarine.

Trans fats are bad fats for your body. It is important to avoid them. The hydrogenation process alters the chemical structure of fats and oils. Through the procedure, hydrogen atoms are added to the oil's double bonds, which enhance the levels of saturated fat and reduce the levels of unsaturated fat. This process prevents rancidity in foods that is caused by the oxidation of fats and oils when exposed to air, light, and moisture.

Manufacturers rely on the use of hydrogenated fats and oils because they increase the shelf life of products considerably. Hydrogenated fats are solid, or partially solid even at room temperature. The hydrogenation process hardens the oils in foods which makes them equally harder for the human body to break down and flush out. Again, it is important to understand product labeling when considering food items. Just because a product is labeled to have "0 grams of trans fat," it is not guaranteed to be completely free of trans fats. In the USA, the FDA allows manufacturers to label a product as "0 grams of trans fat" if it contains less than 0.5 grams of trans fat per serving. Manufacturers take advantage of this leniency in using this label. If you see a product with such a label, the truth is hidden in the list of ingredients. If the product contains less than 0.5 grams of trans fat per serving, you will see the trans fats listed in the ingredients. Eating foods with even a small amount of trans fats on a regular basis can add up to be very bad for your health. With a nutrition certification from Cornell University, this topic is particularly alarming to me. Our societies desperately need to be educated on these facts!

In American culture, having a soda with a crispy pack of potato chips is a common snack habit. It is also common to see people drinking "high energy" soft drinks that carry a promise of boosting energy. Unfortunately, what soft drinks and processed snacks leave behind is a pile of chemicals in your body. They may give you a burst of energy, but at what cost?

I understand that buying canned foods seems to be a convenient way to store foods with a longer shelf life. Many of us find this more of a necessity in the hectic lives we are living. However, canned foods and drinks have preservatives, additives, and dyes or colorants that are not naturally found in food. There is a cost you are paying for convenience.

Chemical-laden foods are like slow poisons that can rot your body from the inside for a long time. The true cost of convenience is revealed when your body can no longer tolerate inflammation and you are faced with other health issues. Detoxification can help you become a smarter and more conscious consumer so that you can choose foods that will improve your health and give you nourishing and lasting bursts of energy.

The moment you begin making the right food choices, you will start leading a life that is more balanced physically, spiritually, mentally, and emotionally. When you go on a mission to clean your diet, you will have to learn to resist the marketing gimmicks and leniencies in the law that make unhealthy foods attractive.

In 1997, the FDA created a new food label that is "Generally

Recognized As Safe" (GRAS). The rule was made to save undue labor that would be needed to review every ingredient in food. The foods that qualify for GRAS can be brought into the market with no verification by the FDA. Companies have abused this rule since its inception and continue to do so today. As a result, there are more than 10,000 chemical additives and preservatives used in food and beverage products.

The way we store food can also transfer contaminants. Plastic containers and wraps are common for food storage, but they pose a potential health risk. The risks of contamination increase when you place plastics in the microwave to heat food. Heat can cause plastic containers to release bisphenol-A (BPA) and phthalates, which are harmful chemicals. Food with higher fat content can pose greater risk of transferring these chemicals when consumed.

Chemicals in plastic containers are endocrine disruptors. They can affect estrogen and testosterone levels in human beings. They can also impact brain growth and the health of reproductive organs in a developing fetus.

The endocrine system is a messenger system in the body that consists of hormones. Endocrine disruptors ruin the communication system in your body. If we think of this in terms of an office, we can relate the endocrine system to the computers and devices that are used for communication. If these devices become infected with a digital virus, they can contaminate all the communication systems for the whole office. This creates chaos because no department can receive messages. Similarly, endocrine disruptors ruin the communication system in your body and spread negativity.

Plastic containers may seem harmless, but BPA can be very harmful, even in low doses. Even plastic cutting boards can contain harmful chemicals. Instead, opt for cooking utensils and containers made of stainless steel, ceramic, or glass. You should avoid using polystyrene cups and takeaway containers. These materials can also release harmful chemicals when exposed to heat. All of these items are damaging to the environment as well as your body.

Aluminum products can also be damaging to health. The human body removes aluminum toxins through urine and feces. However, aluminum can build up over time and eventually damage the nervous system, kidneys, and bones. Heat increases the release of these toxins.

Nonstick pans can also pose a risk to your health. They are very convenient in that they keep foods from sticking during the cooking process. However, the inner coating that makes pans nonstick contains Polytetrafluoroethylene (PTFE). This coating wears away over time. Those particles leach into food and find their way into your gut. The coating can also emit toxic gases and chemicals, even at normal cooking temperatures.

We are constantly exposed to toxic substances. Food is one of the biggest sources of toxins. You can help your body by supplementing it with a clean detox diet. The good news is that you do not have to go on a crash diet or miracle diet in order to implement these practices. A healthy diet can last for a lifetime.

We can CURE THE CAUSES!

Make the decision to eat cleanly and detoxify your body . . . and you will have more energy and feel healthier

CHAPTER THIRTEEN

It's time for delicious detox meals

"What lies behind us and what lies before us are tiny matters compared to what lies within us."

—*Ralph Waldo Emerson*

A DETOXIFYING DIET CAN be delicious and fun! There is no need to feel deprived when you have amazing, healthy options to choose from. Aim for small meal portions and use as few simple ingredients as possible in order to focus on the healthiest foods available. Small portions are easier for your body to process and will give you the maximum nutrient benefits.

Intermittent fasting is a great practice to implement, although it shouldn't be used every day.

The main goal is to minimize exposure to toxic substances and help your metabolism to work better. You will have more energy as you continue to detoxify every day. Each meal of the day will help you get closer to your goal of detoxification.

In this chapter, I have included healthy recipes for breakfast, lunch, dinner, and snacks, as well as juices and dressings. These recipes will equip you to plan every meal of your day to support your overall wellness.

Points to Remember

- Buy organic, non-GMO foods
- Use almond, oat, cashew, macadamia, and coconut flour and milk
- Use olive oil, MCT oil, avocado oil, coconut oil, and grass-fed butter
- Use whole grains
- Limit alcohol intake
- No canned foods
- No nonstick pans; try to use iron or copper
- No plastic cutting boards
- No plastic containers
- No aluminum wraps
- When buying items at the store, check for added sugar and try to limit to five ingredients

Special Note: If you are pregnant, I suggest you consult with your physician before trying any recipe available in this book. Always follow your physician's advice to avoid any complications to yourself and your baby. If you are suffering from a disease and are already under treatment, please consult your physician first. These recipes are just guidelines to get a healthier body inside and out.

Begin your day with a healthy breakfast, the most important meal of the day. Unless you are following a specific diet or fasting, you should make having breakfast a priority. Just like your car cannot start without gas in the tank, the cells in your body cannot function without proper fuel.

Many people may feel that they are too busy for breakfast. If mornings are a busy time for you, plan the night before so you can have a healthy breakfast ready to go. You could even make a quick breakfast of almond milk and espresso or coffee to start your day.

No matter what your schedule is, plan for a great day by starting it off right! Get up, stretch, drink your first glass of water, work out for ten minutes or more, then eat a healthy breakfast. Meditation and stretching can also help rid your body of toxins. Wake up with enough margin of time so that you can prepare and have your breakfast with no rush. Give your body what it needs.

To make the most of your daily food intake, you should schedule your meals just like you schedule all your appointments for the day. You could plan and have healthy foods prepared ahead in your refrigerator or freezer.

I travel, so I try and plan healthy meals for my kids to eat while I am away. I also make sure to pack healthy snacks for myself. Planning is your best tool in making a healthy diet work for you. Remember, you are responsible for creating a healthy lifestyle for yourself. No one else can do this for you. By eating the right foods, you can look and feel better. It is exciting!

Almond Flour Brownies

Ingredients
- 3 eggs
- 150g almond flour
- 2 Tbsp. honey
- Half-cup coconut oil
- 1 Tbsp. vanilla extract
- 75g cocoa powder

- 1/4 tsp. baking soda (optional, not recommended)
- 1/4 tsp. sea salt

Instructions

- Heat the oven to 350 degrees F.
- Put honey, butter, vanilla, and eggs in a bowl and mix until smooth.
- Add almond flour, cocoa powder, baking soda (if used) and sea salt.
- Blend well to make a slightly thick mixture.
- Pour the mixture into the oiled pan and bake for 30 minutes.
- Remove the pan when it is not jiggly anymore and cakey.
- Cool it and cut into a square or rectangular shape for serving.

Almond Butter Cup Cookies

Ingredients

- 1 cup almond butter
- Half-cup of coconut crystals
- 1 tsp. vanilla extract
- ¼ tsp. almond extract
- 2 eggs
- Half-cup almond flour
- 2 tsp. coconut flour

- 100g dark chocolate
- pinch of salt, Himalayan sea salt preferred
- Coconut oil to grease baking sheet

Instructions

- Preheat the oven to 350°F and grease the baking sheet using coconut oil.
- Put almond butter, coconut, vanilla extract, almond extract, and eggs in a bowl.
- Put the almond flour, coconut flour, and salt in a separate bowl and mix.
- Now mix the ingredients of both bowls, and you will have the dough ready.
- Make cookies into the shape of a peanut butter cup. Place them on a baking sheet and bake for 12 minutes until golden. Allow to cool and put in the fridge for half an hour.
- Melt the chocolate, cool it and pour on the top of cookies and place in the fridge until the chocolate turns solid.
- You have delicious cookies ready to be served for breakfast.

Spiced Bran Crackers

Spices make a scrumptious flavor, and this recipe for bran crackers with spices make it an amazing option for breakfast as well as snacks.

Ingredients

- 1 cup all-purpose flour (gluten-free) or coconut flour
- ¾ tsp. coriander (ground)
- ½ tsp. cumin (ground)
- 1⁄4 tsp. chili powder
- 1⁄4 tsp. salt, Himalayan sea salt preferred
- 1⁄4 tsp. black pepper (ground)
- 2 pinches of baking powder
- 1⁄4 cup rice bran
- 1 tbsp. extra virgin olive oil

Directions

- Add flour, rice bran, coriander, chili, black pepper, cumin, salt, and baking powder into a bowl, mix them all and prepare a well in the center.

- Add 3/4-cup water and olive oil, and take a round-bladed knife and move in a cutting motion for mixing until a clump is formed.

- Now knead it with your hands to make a smooth dough.

- Divide the dough into 2 portions, cover and leave for 20 minutes.

- Now roll a portion between 2 sheets of baking paper to form a 2mm thick bread and use a round cutter to cut discs from the bread. Repeat with the other portion. You will have 14- 15 discs in total.

- Heat the oven at 210°C and place all the discs on an oven tray inside and bake for 11 to 12 minutes. Swap trays halfway or until the crackers are browned.
- Leave on the trays to cool down.

You can keep these spiced bran crackers up to 3 weeks in an airtight container which make it an ideal snack for office workers or school going kids, and you can serve them to your guests at teatime as well. This recipe will take some time to prepare, but you can store them for three weeks. Thus, make a jarful of these tasty crackers and enjoy some spare time for a few days.

Herby Omelet

This is a quick and easy to make recipe. It is a wholesome but light meal for breakfast. Herbs make it aromatic and detoxing.

Ingredients

- 2 eggs
- 1½ green onions (finely chopped)
- 1 Tbsp. chives (chopped)
- 1 Tbsp flat-leaf parsley (chopped)
- 1 Tbsp. coriander (chopped)
- ½ Tbsp oregano (chopped)
- Salt to taste, Himalayan sea salt preferred
- 1 tsp. butter

Directions

- Break eggs into a bowl, add a little water and beat well.

- Add all ingredients into the bowl except butter.

- Light the stove on medium heat and melt butter in a pan.

- As the butter melts, pour in the egg mixture and let it cook for 3 to 4 minutes.

- Now fold it in half and serve for eating.

- Avoid overcooking.

- This recipe serves one person. To serve more people, increase the ingredient quantities as per the number of persons to serve.

Almond Flour Crackers

Ingredients

- 100g. almond flour
- 1 egg white
- 1/4 tsp. garlic powder
- 1/4 tsp. onion powder
- pinch of salt

Instructions

- Mix all ingredients and knead to make the dough.
- Now roll it out until it is 1/8-inch thick.
- Cut squares of the rolled-out dough.

- Put on a baking tray and bake at 325°F for 14-15 minutes.
- Check and if they are golden brown, remove from the oven.
- Congrats! You have just made delicious, healthy crackers. This recipe will get you approximately 3 dozen crackers. You can store them in an airtight jar to enjoy the next morning or in your snack time.

Toasty Beans

It is a crispy and light meal and takes less than 10 minutes to prepare, so you do not have an excuse to skip your breakfast.

Ingredients

- 1 Tbsp. olive oil
- 1 Onion (chopped)
- 1 Red chili (chopped)
- 200g mixed and cannellini beans (drained)
- 2 Cherry tomatoes (halved)
- 50ml vegetable stock (homemade)
- 2 Sprigs lemon thyme (no leaves)
- 4 brown bread slices

Instructions

- Heat the oil in a pan, and fry the chopped onion and red chili for 2 minutes.

- Now add beans, tomatoes, stock, and lemon thyme but save a little lemon thyme for garnishing. Cook until the tomatoes begin to cook down.

- Toast the bread slices, sprinkle the beans and remaining thyme on the toasted slices. You are ready to serve your breakfast.

- It is a serving for two persons.

Mushrooms with Toast

Mushrooms are good to fight against inflammation and cancer and help in detoxification.

Ingredients

- 2 eggs
- 10g butter
- 1 onion (diced)
- 1 garlic clove (crushed)
- 1 tomato (Sliced)
- 150g chestnut mushrooms (diced or chopped)
- 1 Tbsp. parsley (chopped)
- 2 toasted bread slices

Directions

- Pour a little water into a pan and boil.

- Break an egg into a cup. Twirl the boiling water and add it in followed by another egg.

- Cook for 2-3 minutes until the egg whites are set and the yolk is still soft. Put the cooked eggs on a dish.

- Melt the butter and fry the onions and garlic for 5 minutes in a pan.

- Increase the flame, add the mushrooms, and cook for another 5 minutes.

- There you go! Now sprinkle mushrooms, eggs, tomato, and parsley on the toasts. Your breakfast is ready.

- It is a serving for 1 person.

Blueberry & Banana Smoothie

Smoothies are nutritious and quick to prepare, and there is a huge variety of smoothies. Also, you can customize the recipes as per your taste. Smoothies make a healthy breakfast. The best thing is that they are free of oil. The following smoothie is a delight for blueberry lovers.

Ingredients

- 250ml almond milk
- 1 small banana
- 1/2 cup blueberries
- 1 Tbsp. ground flaxseed
- 3-4 almonds (flakes)

Directions

- Add all the ingredients to a blender and blend until the mixture is thick and smooth.

- Pour into a glass and enjoy your quick detoxifying smoothie breakfast.

Avocado & Lime Green Tea Smoothie

Ingredients

- ⅔ cup almond milk
- 1 avocado
- ½ lime
- 1 apple (roughly chopped)
- 1 cup brewed, cooled green tea
- A wedge of ginger (peeled)
- ¼ cup parsley
- 2 leaves of kale

Instructions

- Peel all the fruits and cut them into pieces that can fit well into your blender.
- Now add all ingredients into a blender and blend until smooth and your detox smoothie is ready.

Green Tea & Cantaloupe Smoothie

Ingredients

- 1/4 cantaloupe
- 200ml almond milk
- 1/4 cup warm water
- 1½ tsp. green tea powder
- Sugar to taste

Instructions

- Mix warm water with green tea powder to dissolve.
- Add cubed cantaloupe and dissolved green tea powder, sugar, and almond milk in a blender and blend until the mixture is a smooth texture. Enjoy it.

Apple, Cucumber & Mint Smoothie

Ingredients

- 1 apple (green)
- ½ cucumber
- Few mint leaves
- 1 leaf of kale
- Half cup of coconut water
- Half cup cold green tea
- Half lemon

Instructions

- Cut the apples, cucumber, and kale and add to blender with mint, green tea, and coconut water.
- Blend until smooth pour in a glass, then squeeze and mix well before drinking.

Pineapple and Green Tea Smoothie

Ingredients

- 1/4 pineapple (peeled)
- A handful of baby spinach

- Half tsp. green tea powder
- 1 cup of coconut water
- Honey to taste

Instructions

- Add and blend the pineapple and baby spinach leaves in a blender until they are smooth.
- Add green tea powder, coconut water, and honey and mix it well and you are good to go.

Green Punch Smoothie

Ingredients

- 1 cup coconut water
- 1 small mango
- Half-cup pineapple
- 1 tsp. green tea powder
- 1 tsp. ginger paste

Instructions

- Add all ingredients to a blender and blend until your detox green punch detox smoothie is ready.

Almond, Banana, and Date Smoothie

Ingredients

- 1 cup coconut milk
- 5 dates

- 1 banana
- 8-10 almonds (soaked in water overnight)

Instructions

- Remove date seeds.
- Remove almond skins.
- Now add all ingredients into a blender and blend until the mixture is smooth.
- Pour in a glass and enjoy your easy-to-make smoothie.

Coconut, Almond, and Green Tea Smoothie

Ingredients

- 1 cup coconut milk
- 2 Tbsp. almond flour
- 2 bananas (peeled and cut into pieces)
- 2 tsp. green tea powder
- Ice cubes

Instructions

- Put all ingredients into a blender and blend at high speed until the mixture is smooth.
- Pour in a glass and enjoy your smoothie.

Kiwi, Ginger and Green Tea Smoothie

Ingredients

- 2 kiwis (peeled and chopped)

- 1 wedge of ginger (peeled and chopped)
- 1 tsp green tea powder
- 150ml almond milk

Instructions

- Add all the ingredients together in a blender and blend until smooth.

Banana, Spinach, and Kale Smoothie

This green smoothie is a powerhouse of energy and antioxidants. Spinach and kale have antioxidants and help in cleaning body as well as reduce inflammation.

Ingredients

- 1 banana
- 1 cup almond milk
- A handful of spinach and kale
- Ice cubes

Directions

- Blend all the ingredients and add 1 Cup ice if you like to have your smoothie cold.

LUNCH RECIPES

Taking a break during the workday to have lunch is an important practice. You shouldn't skip any meal of the day. Your body needs fuel continuously. If you go too long without eating, you will experience a drop-in energy that can affect the rest of your day. Follow your mealtimes religiously. If you keep your meals lighter, you will be hungry each time you need to eat.

Body detoxification is a lifelong process. You can help your body be more efficient by consuming regular, small meals of organic foods. For midday meals, I recommend soups, salads, and white meats. I have tried my best to share a balanced combination of all types of foods. The following are wonderful ideas for lunches.

Chicken Tenders

Ingredients

- 50g chicken strips
- Half-cup of coconut flour
- 2 eggs
- 2 cups of coconut (shredded)
- 3 Tbsp. coconut oil
- Parsley (chopped)
- Salt to taste

Instructions

- Preheat the oven to 400°F.
- Grease a baking sheet with coconut oil.
- In a dish, mix the coconut flour, cayenne pepper, and salt.
- In a separate dish, break all eggs and whisk well.
- Add coconut in another separate dish.

- Coat all strips in the coconut flour mixture, and dip them in the whisked eggs followed by coating in coconut.

- Now place them on the baking sheet and drizzle them with a little coconut oil.

- Place them in the oven for 15 minutes and flip them over halfway.

- Garnish with chopped parsley, and your crispy chicken tenders are ready. Eat them with yogurt.

Quinoa-Cranberry Grilled Chicken Salad

Ingredients

- 3 large chicken breasts (about 4 lbs.)
- 4 cloves of garlic (chopped)
- 3/4 cup quinoa
- Half-cup scallions (chopped)
- 3/4 cup cranberries (dried)
- 3/4 cup slivered almonds
- 2 Tbsp. olive oil
- 3 Tbsp. apple cider vinegar
- 3 Tbsp. balsamic vinegar
- 1/4 cup lemon juice
- 1 tsp. dried sage
- Sea salt and pepper

Instructions

- Since we will grill the chicken, marinate it overnight for a better taste.

- Slice the breasts into 3 strips.

- Rub the chicken with the chopped garlic, sage, salt, and pepper.

- Place it with 1/4 cup of lemon juice and the apple cider vinegar in a bowl.

- Ensure you cover it and put it in the refrigerator for at least 30 minutes.

- Place the quinoa and 1½ cups of water in a saucepan. Boil and reduce to a simmer and cover. In about 15 minutes, all water will be absorbed by the quinoa. Place quinoa in a bowl to cool completely.

- When the chicken is ready, grill it until it is entirely cooked from the inside as well.

- When the chicken cools down a little, whisk the olive oil, balsamic vinegar, 1 tbsp. lemon juice, and salt and pepper in a bowl. Stir in the chopped scallions to cover them.

- When the chicken is cool to touch, chop into 1-inch cubes. Place the chicken with quinoa, cranberries, almonds, and scallions.

- Add salt and pepper to your own taste.

Roasted Salmon

Ingredients

- 4 pieces of skinless salmon fillet
- 1 Tbsp. vinegar
- 1 Tbsp. seasoning of your choice
- Salt to taste
- Pepper to taste
- 1 Tbsp. ginger (grated)
- 2 tsp. honey
- 2 radishes (cut into half-moons)
- 2 cucumbers (cut into half-moons)
- 1 small onion (sliced)
- A few sprigs of mint (chopped)

Instructions

- Heat oven to 425°F.
- Put the salmon fillets on a pan, brush them well with vinegar, sprinkle the seasoning and salt.
- Roast for 10-12 minutes.
- In the meantime, whisk the ginger, honey, vinegar, salt, and pepper in a bowl, and add the radishes, cucumber, and onion, and mix.
- Serve the roasted salmon on a dish with the salad on the side.

Chickpea, Spinach, and Sausage Stew

Ingredients

- 350g cooked chicken sausage links (sliced)
- 425g chickpeas (rinsed and drained)
- 2 cups of spinach
- 2 cups of chicken stock
- 2 garlic cloves (thinly sliced)
- 200g tomatoes (diced)
- 1 boiled egg
- Salt to taste, Himalayan sea salt preferred
- 2 Tbsp. olive oil
- ¼ tsp. ground black pepper

Instructions

- Take a pan and heat olive oil on a medium flame.
- Now add garlic cloves and simmer for a minute.
- Add chicken sausage links and sauté until they turn golden.
- Add chickpeas, chicken stock, tomatoes, and bring to a boiling point.
- Add spinach, salt, and black pepper and lower the flame to medium and let it cook for 10 minutes.
- Cut the boiled egg in 4 quarters and top it on the stew.
- Your lip-smacking stew is ready to be served. It can be stored in a refrigerator up to 5 days. This recipe can serve 4 persons.

Pumpkin Soup

Ingredients

- 500g pumpkin (peeled and chopped)
- 1 small onion (finely chopped)
- 1 liter of chicken or veggie stock
- 3 cloves garlic (finely chopped)
- 40g smoked tofu (grated)
- 1 Tbsp. of coriander leaves
- ½ Tbsp. olive oil

Instructions

Heat oil in a pan to simmer onion on low flame.

- Now add stock, garlic, and pumpkin, and simmer until pumpkin turns soft.
- Remove it from the stove and pour it into a food processor to puree it.
- Add seasoning to taste and reheat.
- Serve the soup into a bowl topped with tofu, and coriander leaves.
- This recipe can serve 2 persons.

Quinoa Salad

Ingredients

- 1 cup quinoa
- 2 onions
- 1 Tbsp. vinegar

- 1 Tbsp. mustard
- 2 garlic cloves (minced)
- 1 Tbsp. lemon juice
- Salt to taste
- ⅛ tsp. ground black pepper
- ⅛ tsp. cayenne pepper
- 2 tsp. olive oil
- 1 orange
- 1 mango (cut into small cubes)
- 1 cucumber (sliced into half-moons)
- almonds (use another nut if you like)

Instructions

- In a pot, pour two cups of water and bring it to a boiling point.
- Add quinoa and adjust the flame to medium-low and let it cook until liquid is absorbed.
- It will take 5 to 10 minutes.
- Remove the pot and keep it covered for 5 minutes. Now uncover, fluff with a fork, and spread on a platter to let it cool.
- Mix onions, vinegar, mustard, garlic, lemon juice, salt, and black pepper and cayenne pepper, and sprinkle olive oil on it.
- Take the orange, cut, peel, and pith and add to the bowl.

- Now add quinoa, cucumber, mango, and almonds. Mix it softly and sprinkle vinegar on top. Your scrumptious quinoa salad is ready for lunch.

Lentil Salad Tacos

Ingredients

- 2 cups of cooked lentils
- 1 onion (chopped)
- 1 garlic clove (minced)
- A few sprigs of chopped coriander
- 1 avocado (peeled and cut into cubes)
- 1 lime juice
- 2 tsp. olive oil
- 1 tsp. chia seeds
- Salt to taste, Himalayan sea salt preferred
- Ground black pepper
- 2 tortillas

Instructions

- Add lentils, onion, garlic, one teaspoon olive oil, salt, and pepper and mix well. Leave the bowl for 5 minutes.
- Take another bowl and put avocado, parsley, lime juice, and one teaspoon olive oil and mix them well.
- Take a taco, put the lentils and salad on it, sprinkle chia seeds and wrap to serve.

DINNER RECIPES

Dinner signifies to your body that the day is ending. As we complete the day, tiredness may trouble us. We might rush home to enjoy a nice dinner with our family before going to sleep. Your body is tired after a long day and your internal organs are too, including those used in the digestion process. You can give your digestive system and detoxifying organs by having a lighter meal at dinner.

Quinoa Burger

Ingredients

- 1 cup of cooked quinoa
- 1 egg
- 1 onion (diced)
- 1 cup of baby spinach
- 2 garlic cloves (minced)
- Salt to taste, Himalayan sea salt preferred
- Almond oil
- Ground black pepper
- 1 avocado
- 1 lime for juice
- 1 tsp. of chopped coriander
- Whole-wheat bun

Instructions

- Heat the almond oil in a pan, put minced garlic and fry for a minute and put spinach. Let it cook until it the spinach softens and put into a bowl.
- Add quinoa, egg, onion, salt and black pepper in it and mix well.
- Oil the pan with almond oil and fry the bun for a few seconds on each side.
- Put avocado, coriander, and lime juice in the blender to make a smooth paste.
- Halve the bun, apply the paste on the bottom half, put quinoa burger patty, reapply the paste, put one or two onion rings, top it with the other half-bun. Your burger is ready for dinner.

Coconut Oil Roasted Beets

Ingredients

- 2 1/2 pounds beets, peeled and diced
- 2 Tbsp. coconut oil, melted
- 1/2 tsp. coarse salt

Instructions

- Preheat the broiler to 400 degrees.
- Spread the diced beets onto a rimmed heating sheet.
- Sprinkle with coconut oil and hurl to coat all the beets uniformly.
- Include the salt and hurl again to coat with the salt.

- Cook in the preheated broiler for 35-45 minutes or until the beets are delicate or marginally caramelized. Cook them for a longer time if you like firm edges. Be mindful so as not to burn them.

Tuna and Asparagus Salad

Ingredients

- 600g tuna
- 12 spears of asparagus (trimmed)
- 150g salad leaves
- 2 Tbsp. almonds (flaked)
- 1 red chili (seeded and cut into long thin strips)
- 2 green onions (cut into long thin strips)
- Olive oil
- Salt to taste, Himalayan sea salt preferred
- Black pepper
- 1 roasted capsicum
- 1/4 cup coriander leaves

Instructions

- Dip chili and onion in ice-cold water for half an hour and drain.
- Apply a light layer of oil on the pieces of tuna with a brush and rub with sea salt and black pepper.
- Heat a frying pan and sear tuna on all sides until only its surface is cooked, leave the pieces for 10 minutes, and slice into 5mm thick slices.

- Boil water with salt in a pan and blanch asparagus in it for 1 minute, rinse under cold water, and pat dry with an absorbent paper.

- Add chili, onions, asparagus, salad leaves, and capsicum in a bowl and toss softly.

- Put salad mixture in a bowl topped with tuna and almond flakes. The dish is ready to be served.

- This recipe can serve 4 persons. To make a variant of this recipe, replace fish by prawns or quail.

Fish and Prawns with Cucumber

Ingredients

- 200g prawns
- 200g fish fillet
- 1 large cucumber
- 2 tsp. salt
- 4 tsp. olive oil
- 2 cloves of garlic (finely chopped)
- 1 tsp. ginger (grated)
- 2 spring onions (chopped)
- 2 Tbsp. soy sauce
- 1 Tbsp. sesame oil
- Coriander for garnishing

Instructions

- Peel the cucumber, cut it in half, and remove the seeds. Now cut the halves into 1cm or ½ inch slices and sprinkle them with salt. Put them into a colander for twenty minutes to dry.

- Now heat large frying on high flame. Add 2 tsp of olive oil and add the cucumber and stir-fry them until they are of a light brown color. Place them into a serving dish and ensure they are kept warm.
- Add garlic, ginger, and spring onions in the oil and stir-fry them for 30 secs and add fish and prawns and stir fry for 20 minutes.
- Add the soy sauce and sesame oil while stirring carefully for about a minute. Ensure you avoid breaking the fish fillets.
- Now add the cooked fish and prawns to the cooked cucumber.
- Serve in a dish and garnish with coriander leaves.

Winter Chopped Kale Salad with Lemon Vinaigrette

Ingredients

- 1 bunch Lacinato kale
- 3 tablespoons olive oil divided
- 2 Tbsp. lemon juice divided
- 1 cup green cabbage shredded
- 1/2 cup raw beets shredded
- 1/4 cup green scallion chopped
- 1/4 cup parsley chopped
- 1 orange

- 1/2 cup pomegranate seeds
- 1 Tbsp apple cider vinegar
- sea salt and black pepper to taste

Instructions

- Wash, dry and expel the middle ribs from the kale. Shred it finely.

- In an extensive blending bowl, put kale with 1 tablespoon olive oil, 1 tablespoon lemon juice and a touch of salt. Backrub it with your hands for 1-2 minutes or until the kale is splendid green and malleable.

- Include the cabbage, beets, scallions, and parsley and hurl well. Next, include the oranges and pomegranate seeds.

- In a little bowl whisk together olive oil, lemon juice, apple juice vinegar, a touch of salt and pepper. At that point shower the dressing over the plate of mixed greens.

Chicken Veggie Soup

Ingredients

- 3 cups of rotisserie chicken, shredded
- 10-12 cups of chicken stock
- 100g mushrooms, sliced
- 1 onion, chopped
- 4 stalks of celery, chopped

- 2 carrots, peeled & chopped
- 8 cloves of garlic, minced
- ½ tsp. turmeric
- ½ tsp crushed red pepper
- 400g chickpeas
- 2 cups of kale leaves
- 2 Tbsp. olive oil
- Salt to taste

Instructions

- Heat oil over medium-high heat in a big pot and sauté onion, celery, and carrots for 5 minutes.
- Now add mushrooms and garlic and cook for 3-4 more minutes.
- Add the chicken stock, turmeric, red pepper, salt, and chickpeas and bring to a boiling point.
- Now add shredded chicken, cover the pot lower the flame and let it simmer for 20 minutes.
- Add kale leaves, cover the pot and let it simmer for 5 more minutes.
- Your delicious chicken veggie sour is ready for dinner.

Superfood Salad

This recipe can serve 4 to 6 people. It is quick to prepare and takes only 15 minutes. If you are starting to have light meals at dinner, this salad is an ideal choice for you. It will give you a break from heavy meals while it is rich in vitamin and heavily nutritious and delicious.

Ingredients

- 1 small cabbage
- 4 carrots
- 1 beet
- 1 avocado
- ½ cup dill
- 2/3 cup almonds (chopped) Ingredients for Dressing
- 3 garlic cloves
- ½ cup olive oil
- ¼ cup vinegar
- Salt to taste

Instructions

- Shred the cabbage, carrots, and beets in a food processor and put into a bowl.
- Mix pressed garlic cloves, oil, and vinegar to prepare salad dressing.
- Put dill, half of the almonds, vegetables, salt, and the dressing altogether into a bowl and mix them well.
- Taste for salt, and add if needed.
- Sprinkle avocado and remaining almonds on top of the salad and mix it very lightly.
- Your super health super-food salad is ready.

Beef and Broccoli

Ingredients

- 1kg sirloin steak (thinly sliced)
- 1kg broccoli (cut into florets and stalks chopped)
- 2 Tbsp. sesame oil
- 1 cup of water
- 1/4 cup soy sauce
- 3 Tbsp. liquid honey
- 2 Tbsp. cornstarch
- 2 Tbsp garlic (minced)
- 1 Tbsp. ginger (minced)
- 4 green onion (finely chopped)

Instructions

- Whisk 3/4 cup water, soy sauce, honey and cornstarch in a bowl and put it aside.
- Preheat wok on high flame and twirl 1 tbsp. sesame oil for coating. Put beef in it and let it cook until browned a little. When done, put it in a bowl and put the bowl aside.
- Again, swirl remaining sesame oil, add garlic and ginger and cook for half a minute. Put 1/4 cup water and broccoli and keep cook for 2-3 minutes.
- Stir the sauce and add to the wok with beef. Put the flame to medium-low and cook until sauce has thickened.
- Garnish with green onion and eat hot.

Salmon with Spinach and Peas

It is a mouthwatering dish and a treat for salmon lovers. You can serve it in dinner parties as well. This recipe can serve 2 persons.

Ingredients

- 2 salmon fillets
- 400g orange sweet potato (cut into 2cm wedges)
- 1 cup of veggie stock
- 500g peas (podded)
- 1 Tsp. butter
- 2 bunches of spinach
- 2 Tbsp. olive oil

Instructions

- Apply olive oil on sweet potato wedges and roast at 200°C in the oven until they turn brown and tender.
- Bring veggie stock to the boil, add peas and simmer on medium flame until they become tender.
- Drain and reserve stock and refresh peas under cold water.
- Put the peas into a pan, add reserved veggie stock along with butter and mashed peas, and then season to taste.
- Apply oil with a brush on salmon filet and sprinkle salt. Heat a frying pan and simmer the salmon fillets on high flame until they turn brown on both sides.
- In the meantime, put spinach into a pan and cook on medium flame until it is wilted.

- Drain, rinse, and squeeze out excess water, put it back into the pan, season to taste, and toss on the heat with a sprinkle of olive oil.

- Serve wilted spinach in a dish and top with mashed peas and salmon fillets, and place roasted orange sweet potatoes to a side.

SNACK RECIPES

Snacks can easily sabotage your healthy eating plans. Sometimes we snack thoughtlessly. When we do that, we end up making bad food choices. A bag of chips and a soft drink are not healthy snack options.

Eating should not be impulsive. Food cravings make us select foods that are not healthy options. Sometimes we engage in mindless snacking, even when we do not feel hungry.

Sometimes we snack out of habit.

Eating snacks can be an important part of a healthy diet if you plan for them. Steer clear of prepackaged snacks from supermarkets and convenience stores. Have healthy options ready to go. You can even incorporate recipes for cookies, crackers, and brownies shared in the section of breakfast recipes.

Apples

Apples help in digestion and detoxify the body. You can enjoy apples with creamy almond butter to quench your hunger for snacks. It can help in stabilizing blood sugar levels too. You can also eat without any dips, and it will work as finely.

Avocados

Halve an avocado, sprinkle olive oil, lemon juice, and chili pepper to enjoy your snack. It is a highly effective combination of detoxifying agents. Avocados have fiber and antioxidants whereas lemon and olive oil are good for digestion. You can also eat avocado alone since it has fiber, antioxidants, glutathione, and good fats, which make it highly effective for detox. It has a great reputation for weight loss too.

Grapefruit

It is also famous for its weight loss properties as it helps the liver to burn fat. Also, it helps in the treatment of diabetes, makes the body stronger to fight against cancer, and decreases cholesterol levels. It also helps in fighting stomach ulcers, gum diseases, and prevents strokes.

Greek Yogurt

You can accompany Greek yogurt with blueberries that are rich in antioxidants and cinnamon. It makes a power-packed snack with protein and fiber for detoxification.

Pineapple

It is the tastiest detoxifying fruit because of its digestive enzyme called Bromelain, which cleanses the colon. In addition, it balances blood clotting and reduces inflammation.

Watermelon

It has high diuretic effects, so its consumption can make you go to the toilet a little more. It clearly indicates that it helps in removing toxins as toxins pass through urine. Watermelon also helps in regulating blood flow and reduces inflammation and delays the appearance of wrinkles.

Almonds

Almonds are rich in fiber and protein, which remove bowel impurities and balance sugar levels. They are also rich in calcium, magnesium, and vitamin E. A good thing about almonds is that they are easy to carry and can be eaten while working. You can also choose other nuts for snacks.

Blueberries

Blueberries are natural aspirin and possess antiviral properties. Also, they can reduce inflammation and decrease the intensity of pain. They are natural antibiotics and prevent infections in the urinary tract because they block out bacteria. You can keep a handful of blueberries and eat them as a tasty snack.

Green Tea

Green tea is known to work with almost all types of diets, so you can have it with other snacks and meals without any concerns. It is rich in antioxidants and has the ability to remove free radicals in the human body. It is an effective alternative to soda or packaged beverages.

Besides, it has diuretic effects and lowers blood sugar levels.

The next time you want snacks, ensure that you do not tend to pick a pack of snacks from a store, but you have homemade snacks or frits at hand to eat. The good thing is that you do not have to compromise on taste. It is absolutely ok if you cannot replace those unhealthy snacks at once. So, take your time and familiarize your taste buds with organic and detox snacks and you will be right on track to a healthy life.

JUICE RECIPES

The human body consists of 50 to 75% water, which varies depending on the age group and gender. The best purpose water serves in our body is, of course, detox. We lose water through perspiration and urine, which indicates the removal of toxins. Water is itself a detox element, and it can be supplemented with many healthy juices of fruits and vegetables. Thus, take advantage of juices and incorporate them into your daily diet for quicker removal of toxins.

Beetroot, Carrot, and Celery Juice

Beetroot helps your liver in detoxification. Drinking this juice is suitable for breakfast, as a snack, or before dinner.

Ingredients

- 1 beetroot
- 2 carrots
- 2 sprigs of celery
- 3 sprigs of parsley
- A wedge of ginger
- 1 lemon (Optional)

Instructions

- Cut all vegetables and beetroot into small pieces to fit into your juice extractor.
- Process them all together, and you will get your glass of a refreshing, healthy detox juice.
- Squeeze a lemon to enhance flavor.

- Mix it well before drinking.
- It is a serving for one person.

Vegetables with Apple Juice

Green vegetables have chlorophyll, which is a helpful agent for detoxification. It also helps to treat smelly feet, bad breath, and body odor. It is a light and refreshing juice.

Ingredients

- 1 cucumber
- ½ green capsicum (no seeds)
- 3 sprigs of parsley
- 1 green apple

Instructions

- Cut all vegetables and apples into small pieces.
- Process all ingredients together and pour the fresh juice into a glass and enjoy it. If you like, you can add ice cubes.
- It is a serving for one person.

Veggie & Fruit Juice

It is an ideal choice for detoxifying juice as it has lots of green in it.

Ingredients

- 1 carrot
- A small wedge of ginger

- 1 green apple
- ½ lemon
- 1 sprig of celery
- 1 cucumber
- ½ kiwifruit
- ½ cup parsley
- ½ cup sprouts

Instructions

- Cut all ingredients into small pieces.
- Put them in the juicer and pour a glass of cleansing juice into your glass.
- Squeeze the lemon on it and mix it well before drinking.

Tropical Fruit Juice Recipe

It is a healthy and cleansing juice with tropical fruits, and you can enjoy it at breakfast for best results.

Ingredients

- 1/2 pineapple
- 250g papaya (no seeds)
- 1 banana
- Pulp from 1 passion fruit

Instructions

- Cut pineapple and papaya into small pieces and juice them. Put the extracted juice in a blender.

- Add the Banana and blend well and pour into a jug.
- Now stir in the pulp from passion fruit, and you are ready to enjoy a delicious drink.
- You can add lime juice for extra flavor.

Green Detox Juice Recipe

Ingredients

- 1 cup baby spinach leaves
- 1 green apple
- 1 cucumber
- A 1-inch wedge of ginger (peeled)
- 1 small lemon
- Handful parsley leaves with stems

Instructions

- Cut the apple, cucumber, and ginger into small pieces to pass through the juice extractor.
- Peel the lemon, cut into slices, and remove seeds. Put aside about half of the lemon.
- Push all ingredients through the juice extractor and half of the sliced lemon.
- Stir it well and taste for sourness. If it is less sour than your taste, add the remaining lemon.
- If it tastes too sour for you, you can add a carrot.

We can CURE THE CAUSES!

**Eat healthy every
day . . . to support
your overall wellness**

CHAPTER FOURTEEN

Are you ready to go shopping the detox way?

"An apple a day keeps the doctor away."

—*Welsh Proverb*

S HOPPING THE DETOX way is essential to leading a healthy lifestyle. It is important to understand that detox not only applies to you as a person but also to the environment in which you live.

To put it simply, no matter how clean you are, you cannot be healthy if the house you are living in is full of toxins and vice versa. This mentality will help you shop consciously to ensure that you have what you need to eliminate toxins from your body and your home. You must arm yourself in the fight against toxins!

There are important things that you need to keep on hand to help you in the process of detoxification. Just as your house cannot be cleaned without the right cleaning agents, your body cannot detoxify without the right ingredients. When they run out, you must replace them just as you would replace the cleaning products for your home.

Healthy food should be at the top of your "detox" shopping

list. Food is a very important part of daily life. Toxins enter your body through the food you consume. Thus, it is extremely important to consume healthy and toxin-free foods. Make it a point to buy only those foods and plan your diet in a manner that will aid the detoxification process rather than cause a disturbance to it.

Various foods can help in the process of detoxification. Your health depends on the kinds of food you buy and consume. When you go shopping, it is vital that you buy fruits and green vegetables. These foods are essential to the process of detoxification. Fruits help our bodies to remove toxins because they have a high percentage of water content. This aids the body's internal cleansing system in washing away toxins. Fruits also contain important vitamins and minerals that help the body's defense system fight off toxins.

Citric acid is an important substance that is found in citrus fruits such as lemons, oranges, and limes. Citric acid helps the body remove many toxins. It also aids in digestion by providing helpful enzymes that break down food. Lemon juice is particularly beneficial to the liver, kidneys, and other organs responsible for the internal cleansing process. Lemon juice can make the detoxification process more efficient. In fact, I recommend that you begin your mornings with a warm glass of lemon water.

Green vegetables play a vital role in making sure the body is constantly shielded from toxins in the environment. I always recommend that people buy and eat as many green vegetables as possible. One reason that green vegetables are so important in detoxifying is the chlorophyll they contain. Chlorophyll rids the body of harmful environmental toxins such as heavy metals and toxins that might be present in herbicides, pesticides, and cleaning products. Chlorophyll aids the liver in thoroughly removing toxins from the body.

One unique vegetable that is very beneficial for detoxification is garlic. Garlic can help your body rid itself of many toxic elements. It also aids the liver in producing detoxifying enzymes that filter toxic elements from the digestive system. You can easily add sliced or cooked garlic to your food as a part of a detox diet.

Other foods that are beneficial for detoxification are onions, carrots, artichokes, asparagus, broccoli, cabbage, kale, Brussels sprouts, cauliflower, beets, turmeric, and oregano. These foods can provide a great base for a healthy, nutritious, and detoxifying diet. They can be eaten cooked, juiced, or raw. In combination, these foods can aid the liver in removing waste and harmful toxins. These foods also have a large amount of naturally occurring sulfur that supports liver function and strengthens the body against toxins in the environment.

Seeds and nuts are other natural ingredients that can benefit our health. Flaxseed, pumpkin seeds, almonds, walnuts, hemp seeds, sesame seeds, chia seeds, Siberian Cedar nuts, and sunflower seeds are all very helpful to our bodies in fighting off toxins. Nut butters can be a great way to add nuts to your diet; just be sure to avoid products with added sugars and hydrogenated oils as these can end up doing more damage than good.

Green tea is another natural substance that can aid in the process of detoxification. Green tea has many properties that help the body eliminate toxins. It also has a naturally occurring material that helps the liver to act in a more efficient manner. Green tea supports the function of the liver that allows it to completely remove toxins from the body and help it stay cleaner and healthier.

Beans are also very helpful in the detoxification process. There are numerous kinds of beans, but the most important is Mung beans. Mung beans are highly nutritious and have been used by medical practitioners for thousands of years. They are easy to digest and are known to absorb toxins that remain in the intestinal walls. They are readily available, so you should add these to your shopping list.

Healthy foods such as fruits and vegetables should be considered a gift to us from nature. You should make sure to buy them as often as possible. Plan meals that utilize healthy, fresh ingredients and prioritize your budget to make buying healthy food a top priority.

There is no way to completely avoid toxins. There are simply too many ways they can enter our systems through food, water, secondhand smoke, vehicle emissions, chemical spills, pesticides, and pollution. Even stress can serve as a toxin that can harm our bodies.

Maintaining a diet that is high in detoxifying foods is one of the best ways to keep your body healthy and strong. However, even the best diet cannot completely block toxins from entering your body. In order to combat this, I recommend following the Body Cleanse Diet. This will aid in the removal of any toxin that manages to enter your system before it is able to cause any harm to your organs.

The first step to any full body detox is a thorough colon cleanse. This is only possible through the intake of food that has a high amount of fiber in it. Fiber can make your colon cleaner by helping to remove toxic waste and other harmful elements through your stool. This will help your body to remain free of any substances that can cause harm to it.

As you make detoxification a priority in your life, you will want to consider every purchase you make in relation to the positive or negative effects it can have on your health. Purchasing decisions regarding personal care products cannot only affect your wallet, but also your health. Unfortunately, it is almost impossible to find beauty and personal care products that do not contain any toxic chemicals.

Often the biggest concern in buying personal care products is how quickly they can make us look better. We often don't consider the effects these products can have. In truth, personal care products can be very harmful to your skin and overall health.

Many products that are categorized as "makeup" have a huge number of toxins. Please do not waste your money on products that are harmful to your health in the name of beauty. Chemicals found in beauty products can be very detrimental.

If you read the list of ingredients on many beauty products available today, you will find many of the following chemicals including phthalates, lead, Quaternium-15, and toxin-releasing preservatives such as PEG compounds, BHT, BHA, parabens, Octinoxate, carbon black, and siloxanes. There are many more, but these are a few that you should be aware of that can cause damage to the body.

Phthalates are a group of chemicals that are known to cause damage to the endocrine system, which is responsible for the release and production of hormones. Certain chemicals can lead to reproductive and neurological toxins that may cause permanent damage to organs. Phthalates are used in the manufacturing of plastic products. They make products more flexible and better able to carry color and smell.

Even if phthalates are not listed on the ingredients list, they may still be present in products as manufacturers often try to group such chemicals under the heading of "fragrance." Some companies consider their fragrance formula to be a trade secret. In this way, they are not fully disclosing to the consumer what their product contains. I recommend avoiding all products that have the generic term "fragrance" listed as an ingredient. It is better to choose products that utilize natural plant oils instead.

Lead is also widely used in beauty and skincare products. It is considered one of the most dangerous elements for the human body. As such, it is usually categorized as a "neurotoxin."

Neurotoxins are highly poisonous substances to the nervous system that can lead to miscarriages, reduced fertility, and can even delay the onset of puberty in females.

To find lead in your beauty store, you probably need to look no further than the selection of lipsticks. Artificial colors very commonly contain lead. Each time you use lipstick, you could be allowing lead to enter your body. Ironically, if you are following a detoxification regimen, you may not even need to use lipstick because your natural coloring will come through. I highly recommend that you discontinue the use of any product that contains lead.

Parabens are also very dangerous to human health and widely used as chemical preservatives in cosmetics and other products. They are highly dangerous because they can penetrate the skin very easily and enter the bloodstream. They can cause serious damage to the body's defense system. They have also been detected in human breast cancer tissue. I do not think it is a coincidence that as the use of products with dangerous chemicals has increased, so has the number of females suffering from breast cancer.

Quaternium-15 is another toxic chemical that is used in cosmetics such as mascara, pressed powders, and eyeliners. This chemical can cause skin problems and irritation. I believe it to be a skin cancer-causing chemical.

I am including information about these dangerous chemicals to increase consumer awareness. These elements are present in products we all use daily. Shopping in the detox way will change the way you make purchase decisions. You will be more conscious of what is acceptable to you. Make the choice to use more natural products that are beneficial, instead of harmful to your health.

It will take time for you to adjust to these changes. Making fruits and vegetables a greater part of your diet will become second nature. You will begin to acquire a taste for them. Consider it a challenge and watch how your body adapts and responds positively to healthy changes.

Detoxification is about facing your fears and your weaknesses and eliminating them. Make it your goal to avoid using all products that can harm your health. It is a tough job, but your organs need all the help you can give them. This is exactly what shopping the detox way looks like. Let your hard-earned dollars be your voice in refusing to purchase foods and products that contain highly toxic elements. Instead, support the producers of healthy, natural foods and products. It is a great challenge, but you can do it. The International Science Nutrition Society sends out a monthly newsletter that can help you can stay up to date on many scientific ways to detox the body through your diet.

We can CURE THE CAUSES!

**Prioritize your budget
to make buying organic
healthy food a top priority**

CHAPTER FIFTEEN

Adopting the detox lifestyle for a lifetime

"When you arise in the morning think of what a privilege it is to be alive, to think, to enjoy, to love."

—*Marcus Aurelius*

T HE DETOX LIFESTYLE is not something you can follow for just a few days in order to get results. This way of life is for keeps! You have the power and information you need to adopt this way of life for your entire lifetime. Begin making changes, one by one. It will get easier every day and become a way of life that you can maintain throughout your lifetime.

The battle is half won just by knowing the root causes of your health issues. This knowledge will make preventive measures more important to you. Before long, you will be doing more and more to detoxify yourself and the environment.

Our bodies are gifts from God. Yet, these gifts are only temporary. Someday, we will each face death. We should not take our time on earth for granted. Instead, we should make the most of each day by maintaining our health with all the resources we have available.

Some people may consider investing in a healthy lifestyle a waste of time and money. It is up to us to decide what is most important to us. Money can buy many things, but it cannot buy back health once it is destroyed.

Some people will still choose to live a life full of toxic substances, despite knowing the harms they can cause. They will completely ignore the truth and keep on doing what they have always done. Eventually, the level of toxicity in their bodies will become so high that they will begin to experience negative symptoms.

Throughout this book, I have been asking the question, "Why are we not working to cure the causes of disease?"

Our healthcare system of today is reactive. When we have a reactive approach to health, we are forced to deal with consequences. We lose the opportunity to focus on precautions. I am a proponent of more proactive measures in healthcare. These measures take a stand against all the toxins that are present in our environment. Instead of allowing these toxins to cause various kinds of diseases, we must eliminate them at all costs.

The toxins that we face in our environment are stronger than ever. I cannot overstate the potential damage that can be done by these toxins. We are beginning to see high blood pressure, diabetes, and other diseases as the "norm." These conditions do not have to be our fate. We do not have to rely on prescriptions and procedures. We can instead revolutionize our lifestyles!

I travel the world speaking about the importance of a healthy body and the ways in which optimum health can be achieved. I always stress the importance of making our lives toxin-free. It will require some very big changes to our diet and routine. Most of all, we need to change our mindset. We need to understand the importance of a healthy and disease-free life.

Detoxification is one of the most important changes we can implement. Detoxification is the best way to protect ourselves and our children from the toxic environment. This process must be done continually throughout our lives.

Even though detoxification will require a commitment to some pretty big changes, in the long run, you will be thankful. Detoxification can help you avoid life-long dependency on medications. It can even help you prevent pain and debilitation. Results will not happen overnight. Over time, by keeping with the detoxification lifestyle, you will strengthen your body against the harmful elements that may try to enter. Your body's natural defenses will be at the ready to withstand toxins.

The reason that detoxification has become so important to optimal health in modern times, is that humankind has chosen a path of destruction in recent decades. Generations before us enjoyed an atmosphere and environment that was clean and healthy. They were also more physical in their daily lives, which made their bodies tougher and stronger.

As the human lifestyle has evolved into a sedentary one, physical fitness and resilience have declined. The effects of this are compounded by the increased toxins within our environment. It is further compounded by the chemicals we put into our bodies through food and exposure to common household items. We are dependent on the very things that are making us weaker—our technology and our conveniences. These things are not only weakening us, but they are also poisoning us.

Today, we want to achieve everything without doing anything. The importance of hard work is minimized. The youth of today do not understand that nothing is ever achieved without passion and hard work.

To help explain the importance of hard work, I want to

bring attention to an example in nature. A butterfly emerging from its cocoon is an everyday miracle. I want you to think of this process in your mind. A butterfly does not hatch out of its cocoon in one easy motion. When it begins to emerge, it creates a small opening. The butterfly must work very hard to push itself out of the cocoon little by little. This difficult process is vital to the butterfly's survival. The process of emerging from the cocoon is nature's way of forcing blood into the butterfly's newly formed wings. Without this process, the butterfly will not be able to use its wings and fly.

Human beings require struggle in order to find their capabilities, just like a butterfly must struggle from its cocoon in order to be able to fly. If we want to achieve our maximum potential, we must work hard for it. The trials and challenges will make us stronger.

This principle applies to detoxification as well. It is something we must work hard for, but the process will make us stronger. Detoxifying your body is a regular exercise that can produce amazing results. The toxins in our world are stronger than ever. We must be stronger than ever in order to fight them! This is something you need to do for yourself and all of the people in your life.

If you are a parent, this process is even more important for you. Your children need you. You must be strong for them physically, emotionally, and spiritually. I urge parents to take their health very seriously. Being a parent is indeed a blessing. This blessing should never be taken for granted. I urge you to begin this process of body detoxification now so that you can be there for your children and serve as an example for them to live by.

As you implement detoxification into your own life, it is important to further awareness about the importance of detoxification for those around you. Many people do not adopt a healthy lifestyle because they are not aware of the benefits. The concept of detoxification is very new.

Now that you have this knowledge, you can help to share the message.

Even the most health-conscious people are still consuming many unhealthy items. They are unaware of the harmful effects of the toxins they are exposed to. The detox lifestyle can help anyone to cleanse their body and tackle the problem of toxic overload. Even if you are not able to eliminate toxins from your body and the environment, a few simple steps can have very positive effects. Consistency can make small changes in your life have tremendous power.

One of the most important things you can do is increase your fiber intake. The organs that are responsible for the filtration of toxins from the body depend on fiber. If you include plenty of fiber in your daily diet from organically produced fresh vegetables and fruits, your body will be able to function at its best.

Radishes, artichokes, broccoli, cabbage, parsley, grapefruit, and beets are vegetables that are extremely high in fiber. Eating those foods while avoiding processed foods, caffeine, alcohol, and refined sugars will produce optimum results.

You can also remove toxins from your skin and ensure improved blood circulation through daily oil massages and skin scrubbing. You can dry-brush and take baths to remove toxins from your pores. Before taking a shower, you can dry brush your body. These practices will improve blood circulation and promote the elimination of toxins through the skin. The apparel line coming from ABC's For Life will also assist with this process by simply wearing the garments! They have even developed an animal line that protects your pets and livestock from toxins!

Drinking water is also very important for your health. Water is a catalyst for all the detoxification methods that are presented in this book. Staying hydrated will allow your body to be able to flush away toxins. The more hydrated you are, the more toxins you can remove from your body. Make sure it is filtered water, however, as our water contains many natural and chemical contaminants. I could write an entire chapter on this topic, but may save that for next time. Simply said, quality water is imperative to your health and life.

Hydrotherapy can be highly effective. There are many ways to do this. One simple way is to swap between hot and cold water during a shower. Take a hot shower for a couple of minutes and then turn to cold water for about three seconds. Repeat this process three times, then lay down for about thirty minutes. The hot water helps to dilate your blood vessels. The cold water contracts your blood vessels. The change between the two is useful in reducing inflammation and eliminating toxins from the tissues. This can aid in overall circulation.

All of these are small things that you can implement quickly. I want to also mention the effects of alcohol consumption on the body. More than 90-percent of alcohol is processed in the liver. The liver secretes various chemicals that convert alcohol into a potentially cancer-causing chemical called acetaldehyde.

Acetaldehyde is a chemical compound that is linked to most of the negative clinical effects of alcohol. The liver converts acetaldehyde into a harmless substance called acetate and it is later eliminated from the body. Various studies have shown that the consumption of alcohol can cause various kinds of health problems. Excessive consumption can damage your liver function to a great extent by causing increased amounts of fat and inflammation. When this happens, your liver cannot function properly and perform the task of filtering waste and other toxins. Abstaining from alcohol is one of the best ways to keep your body's natural detoxification system running strong.

The most important thing to remember is that your body is a complete package. Habits related to your health should be made from a holistic approach considering mind, body, and spirit as one. In addition to detoxifying physically, you should make a point of letting go of negative thoughts and feelings. Let go of grudges and be welcoming to others. Negativity can break down your spirit, which is what gives your body life. If you hold on to negativity, you will soon be left with nothing but regrets. Embrace peace, love and happiness!

Life is a long journey. I hope you will make the decision to take care of your health so that you can live your best life. Bring others along in your journey. Celebrate wellness together as a way of life. Love the life you have by making it the life you deserve!

We can
revolutionize our lifestyles

We can
CURE THE CAUSES!

CHAPTER SIXTEEN

Dr. Christina Rahm's web-based education courses

I HAVE A MASTER'S of Science in Rehabilitation Science, Doctorate Degrees in Counseling Psychology and Strategic Science, and have done post-doctoral work in Nanobiotechnology and Bioscience Engineering, and have received certificates in Nutrition and Pharmaceutical Management. I am a great advocate of technological advancement and have dedicated my life to study, research, and formulate products that can better the environment and help us all live longer, healthier lives. It is my mission to bring others alongside me on this journey to wellness. I am currently offering a selection of web-based education courses at www.drchristinarahm.com designed to broaden understanding of how nutraceuticals can benefit humanity and the earth.

CLASS 1: INTRODUCTION TO NUTRACEUTICALS

Learn about nutraceuticals, dietary supplements, fortified foods, functional foods, and nutraceuticals and the roles they play in the pharmaceutical and medical food industries globally.

CLASS 2: CONCEPT, BIOCHEMISTRY OF NUTRITION AND DIETETICS

Learn to classify food components based on their nutritional value and how to conduct a nutritional assessment of carbohydrates, proteins, and fats to formulate recommended dietary intake. This course also contains in-depth studies of acceptable dietary intake, nitrogen balance, protein efficiency ratio, and net protein utilization. Students will also learn the basics of energy balance in relation to basal metabolic rate (BMR), body mass index (BMI), and standard dynamic action (SDA) with special reference to nutraceuticals.

CLASS 3: NUTRITION RELATED DISEASES AND DISORDERS

Excess and deficiencies of carbohydrates, protein, amino acids, fat, vitamins, and minerals can be linked to certain diseases and chronic conditions. Learn how these elements, as well as the use of nutraceuticals, can contribute to the prevention and management of diseases such as diabetes mellitus, hypertension, hypercholesterolemia, and cancer. You will also learn about the use of antioxidants as dietary supplements to prevent and treat cancer, obesity, and stress. This course will also explore the role of nutraceuticals and functional foods as they relate to pediatrics, geriatrics, sports performance, pregnancy, and lactation.

CLASS 4: NUTRACEUTICALS OF PLANTS

In this course, you will learn about plant secondary metabolites; their classification, and sub-classification into Alkaloids, phenols, and Terpenoids. You will also learn about the extraction and purification of plant secondary metabolites and their applications. Specific examples will be explored in reference to skin, hair, eye, bone, muscle, brain, liver, kidney, and general health improvements and stimulants. The concepts of cosmeceuticals and aquaceuticals will be introduced.

CLASS 5: NUTRACEUTICALS OF ANIMAL ORIGIN

Nutraceuticals of animal origin have many uses and applications in preventive medicine and treatment. This course will explore sources and extraction of animal metabolites, including chitin, chitosan, glucosamine, chondroitin sulfate, and other polysaccharides, and how they contribute to human health and wellness.

CLASS 6: MICROBIAL AND ALGAL NUTRACEUTICALS

In this course, students will gain an understanding of prebiotics and probiotics and their many applications as related to human health and wellness. Students will learn the principle, mechanisms, production, and technology involved. Examples of bacteria used as probiotics and prebiotics in maintaining useful microflora will be explored as well as their extraction from plant sources. Other topics will include the use of synbiotics for maintaining good health and the extraction and enrichment of algae as a source of omega-3 fatty acids, antioxidants, and minerals.

About The Author

Dr. Christina Rahm is an internationally sought-after scientific leader, spokesperson, and innovator in health and wellness today. She travels the world presenting, lecturing, and educating the private and public sectors about the bold new world of nutraceuticals, wellness strategies, and environmental solutions. She has given lectures for Johns Hopkins Continuing Medical Education among many others.

Dr. Rahm has masters and doctorate degrees in Rehabilitation Counseling Sciences Psychology, and Strategic Science. She has conducted postdoctoral studies at Harvard University in Bioscience Engineering and Nanobiotechnology, and received certificates in Nutrition, and Pharmaceutical Management from Cornell University. She has served in positions like Chief Scientific Officer, Chairman of the Board of Medical Sciences and Clinical Sciences, spokesperson and lab formulator for companies such as Pfizer, Johnson & Johnson, Jansen, DCZ Healthcare, Biogen, Idec, Alexion, Rain International, and Root Wellness.

Invited to speak all over the world, she shares from her personal experience as a cancer and Lyme disease survivor where she faced life and death choices while pregnant with twins. She bravely chose to follow her heart, taking her health and wellness into her own hands instead of following the traditional course of treatment. She has brought many of the products she has made to the world through Root Wellness, and ABC's For Life.

Dr. Rahm has channeled her passion as a visionary in health and wellness into creating multiple provisional patents and proprietary formulas. Her focus is on developing natural products from a holistic approach of curing the causes of disease through detoxification of the body and the environment. Her mission is "to love, empower, and help others to be the best they can be through education on health and wellness."

She has developed several consulting programs for life and wellness that assess personal and professional strategies to help people attain optimum emotional, mental, and physical health and live longer and more productive lives. Clients' benefit by gaining clarity through the process of mental road-mapping that detoxifies the mind and spirit.

Dr. Rahm is dedicated to caring for the environment and utilizes her experience working in environmental detox engineering to offer her "Environmental Awareness" program and "Environmental Clean-up Consulting" program that focuses on detoxifying homes and property and making the air, land, and water cleaner for everyone.

Her holistic approach offers "Relationship Health Consulting" and "Friendship Coaching" that focus on dating, marriage, sexual health, and relationships. Her program helps people navigate the complexities of contemporary family life and the challenges of building new relationships while strengthening old ones.

Dr. Rahm also offers a "Corporate and Personal Wellness Consulting" program that provides individualized strategies for personal development in the corporate sector. In 2021, she will launch the Dr. Christina Rahm brand of solutions for health, wellness, and life, with the release of this book, "*Cure the Causes*."

References

AMERICAN CANCER SOCIETY. Key Statistics for Lung Cancer. October 1, 2019. https://www.cancer.org/cancer/small-cell-lung-cancer/about/key-statistics.html

ASTHMA UK. "Asthma Facts & Statistics." (n.d.) https://www.asthma.org.uk/about/media/facts-and-statistics/

BREASTCANCER.ORG. "U.S. Breast Cancer Statistics." February 13, 2019. https://www.breastcancer.org/symptoms/understand_bc/statistics

CDC, Smoking & Tobacco Use, "Current Cigarette Smoking Among Adults in the United States," CDC, February 4, 2019, https://www.cdc.gov/tobacco/data_statistics/fact_sheets/adult_data/cig_smoking/index.htm.

CENTER FOR FOOD SAFETY, "Are GMOs Safe? No consensus in the science, scientists say in peer-reviewed statement. CFS. February 19, 2015. https://www.centerforfoodsafety.org/press-releases/3766/are-gmos-safe-no-consensus-in-the-science-scientists-say-in-peer-reviewed- statement

EWG. "Body Burden: The Pollution in Newborns." Environmental Working Group, July 14, 2005. https://www.ewg.org/research/body-burden-pollution-newborns

INTERNATIONAL SCIENCE NUTRITION SOCIETY. (ISNS). www.sciencenutritionsociety.com

FEDERAL REGISTER. Food Labeling: Trans. "A Rule by the Food and Drug Administration. July 11, 2003. https://www.federalregister.gov/documents/2003/07/11/03-17525/food-labeling- trans

STATISTA. Consumer Goods & FMCG Food & Nutrition. "Worldwide sales of organic food from 1999 to 2017 (in billion

U.S. dollars)." M. Sahbandeh. August 9, 2019. https://www.statista.com/topics/1047/organic-food-industry/

STATISTA. Global spending on medicines 2010-2023. "Global spending on medicines in 2010, 2018, and a forecast for 2023 (in billion U.S. dollars)." Mikulic, Matej, August 27, 2019. https://www.statista.com/statistics/280572/medicine-   spending-worldwide/

THE CHALKBOARD. "Sweat Therapy: 6 Detoxifying Workout Routines To Do On (Or Off) Your Juice Cleanse." Horwich, Katie, January 8, 2015. https://thechalkboardmag.com/sweat-therapy-6-detoxifying-workout-routines-juice-cleanse

United States Department of Agriculture. "Establishing the National Bioengineered Food Disclosure Standard." USDA. December 20, 2018https://www.usda.gov/media/press- releases/2018/12/20/establishing-national-bioengineered-food-disclosure-standard

University Health News—DAILY. NUTRITION. "10 Natural Detox Foods & Nutrients to Protect Your Child from Toxins." Staff, UNF, September 5, 2013. https://universityhealthnews.com/daily/nutrition/10-natural-detox-foods-nutrients-to-protect- your-child-from-toxins/

Endorsements

"I have had the privilege of knowing Dr. Rahm for a number of years. Being an internationally acclaimed research scientist who has contributed to numerous innovations in the fields of medical and clinical science, we have also had the opportunity to work together in multiple international projects aimed at improving health, wellness, nutrition and overall quality of life for people throughout the world. Her education includes Masters, Doctorate, and post-graduate work in various areas of science that were earned from public, private, international and Ivy League colleges and universities over the last 30 years of her life. Additionally, having worked for some of the top medical and clinical science pharmaceutical biotechnology companies in the world as well as some of the top nutrition and nutraceutical supplement companies, Dr. Rahm has had exposure in almost every area of healthcare. She has been able to assist people, governments, companies and societies by traveling to over 70 countries where she has educated and provided solutions to some of the most acclaimed members of these communities. After getting to know Dr. Rahm, I was able to understand that her dedication and devotion to health and wellness, stems from her true passion and love for her family, her friends, and even those she has never met. Her lack of fear in working all over the world, comes from her need to heal and serve others. She is not just an expert in the field of health and wellness, she has dedicated her life to the advancement of others, even in her ability to work and serve in 3rd world countries. It is hard to believe the amount of work and energy she has put into her life's mission, but as I have worked with her, I have begun to understand that, to her, this stems from her life's calling to help others. I wish I could say that her path has been smooth, but, the truth is, anyone trying to make changes for the betterment of others, experiences attacks and criticism. Being a leader, she has put herself on the front line, knowing that controversy will occur, but with the knowledge that she owes it to others to advocate for better approaches in healthcare. I celebrate her knowledge and commitment to improvements in others' lives. Cure the Causes is a "must- read" for anyone wanting to improve their path to wellness and improvement in their lives. The book can be a start to a positive change for many people, and for many companies."

—**Kline Preston** is an attorney, author, and entrepreneur that lives in Nashville, Tennessee. He represents numerous celebrities, athletes, musicians, and politicians, and has been involved in numerous health and wellness endeavours throughout his career. He is an acclaimed international attorney that has served as an election observer in three Russian elections: the 2011 Parliamentary Elections, the 2012 Presidential Elections and the 2016 Parliamentary Elections. In 2012 he was the Chairman of the Independent Foreign Election Observers for the Presidential Election. He has been awarded the Nikolai Girenko Award for his contributions to Russian Civil Law. Additionally, in 2014, Mr. Preston was awarded the Order of the Russian Nation for his contributions to Russian-American relations by the Russian Senate.

"My friend, Christina Rahm, or rather Dr. Christina Rahm, as she is professionally known, is absolutely brilliant. I would recognize this perspective more than most as we have been close friends since elementary school. Christina is remarkably intelligent with a whirlwind of resolve as she has overcome much in her life including multiple cancer diagnoses and personal trauma. I have listened to her discuss the importance of needing to 'Cure the Cause' for many years. I too have undergone health-related consequences due to a diagnosis of breast cancer and hospital-acquired infections. I have learned so much from Christina on the importance of detoxification to support healing; I hope you will too."

—**Lisa Crites** is the award-winning inventor of The SHOWER SHIRT®, the first and only patented, a water-resistant garment to protect chest surgery patients while showering. Following her breast cancer diagnosis and double mastectomy surgery in 2009, Lisa was reduced to showering in a plastic trash bag to protect her surgical drain sites. Subsequently, she designed, manufactured, and now distributes The SHOWER SHIRT® both nationally and internationally, to post-mastectomy and chest surgery patients. The product has been exported to patients in Canada, England, Ireland, Israel, Australia, New Zealand, Japan Austria, Dubai, Spain, Portugal, Cyprus, and Seychelles.

Lisa was awarded the 2015 InnovateHER winner for The SHOWER SHIRT® for the Southeast Region of the US and placed 2nd in Washington DC for the National InnovateHER series sponsored by the SBA, Washington Post, and Microsoft. Lisa received a 2015 Patient Innovation award from the University of Portugal, School of Business & Economics, and recently requested by Dubai ruler, King Sheik Mohammad, to present at the World Government Summit—Edge of Government exhibit in the United Arab Emirates. Additional international honors include a 2016 request from the London Science Museum to host The SHOWER SHIRT® for the museum's Science Innovation exhibit.

She has been featured in both FORBES Magazine and the Huffington Post; FOX News, CBS, NBC, CNN, and Lifetime TV's, 'The Balancing Act,' discussing her invention and the legislative filing of the 'Post Mastectomy Infection Reduction Act,' sponsored by Congressman Bill Posey (R-FL) and Congressman Debbie Wasserman-Schultz (D-FL). A Broadcast Journalist, Corporate Healthcare Consultant, Media Strategist, guest speaker, print columnist, blogger, and entrepreneur, Lisa has more than 27 years of experience in the fields of health/medical journalism and news issue/crisis management.

"We never forget how it felt like to meet Dr. Christina Rahm for the first time. It was like in a center of a Hurricane, when you can see the endless energy all around you but In the middle of it it is just smart, and calm wholeheartedness. She is an absolutely devoted professional, activist, and a great doctor who would always be there for you. Knowledge and perseverance, that is her as well, and of course a great author, so congratulations on her new book!"

—**Dr. Norbert Ketskes M.D.** general practitioner, nutritionist, celebrity and Olympic athlete healthcare specialist, and his wife Dr. Zsuzsa Csisztu, former Olympic medalist, sport-lawyer, member of the Hungarian Olympic Committee, and award-winning actress.

"I have had the privilege of knowing Dr. Christina Rahm on a personal and professional level for the last several years. She has a special gift that she has shared around the world, while at the same time be an amazing mother to her four beautiful children. While her ivy league education and knowledge in her field are impressive, it's her heart to help others that I have come to admire. Her healing energy, depth of knowledge, and desire to help others heal, draws people to her wherever she goes. I believe Dr. Christina is a modern-day alchemist and this book will be life-changing to so many who are in need of healing and optimal health."

—**Joy Smallwood**, is a mother of three and an internationally acclaimed photographer having worked and traveled the world with numerous celebrities, models and corporations. Joy has worked with Dr. Rahm professionally and has also known her personally for many years through their children.

"Dr Christina Rahm, through her life's story, shows extraordinary tenacity in the face of adversity which has forged not only a courageous human being but a unique approach to life itself."

—**Clare G. Harvey**, CEO Floweressence CGH (Dip Shen Tao) is an internationally recognized Harley Street Consultant, formulator, inventor, and author of seven books in the field of complementary and integrative medicine. A third generation Bach expert, she is known for her pioneering work and eclectic approach with Flower Essences and their ability to address the root cause of disease and disharmony. Co-founder of Adaptofleur, body organ targeted flower remedies as well as co-creator of the first-ever Floragex: Nordic Flower Essence Line.

"I had the pleasure and opportunity to work and create amazing dialogue with Dr. Rahm on Episode #060 of the Healthcare360 podcast. I am a genuine fan of Dr. Rahm's work, and how she is atypical in her thorough approach to healthcare at large!

Dr. Rahm is an inspiration of hope to others by providing them unparalleled knowledge matched with an empathetic caring heart . . . This is the new model of Healthcare, and it's right in front of us."

—**Scott E. Burgess**, founder and owner of Healthcare360 Media, LLC, which has been nominated and voted as one of the best Healthcare podcasts of 2020, TWICE!

"As a businesswoman whose career ended earlier because of health complications due to the 9/11 terrorist attack, I've had to keep my health and wellness at the forefront of my life. Being the mom of three very active boys, it's very important for me to stay as healthy as possible. Since meeting Dr. Christina Rahm, she has guided me and helped navigate my health care plan to assist me in finding the healthiest natural solutions for improving my health. I have trusted her with critical decisions in regards to keeping me as healthy as possible and she has surpassed all expectations. As I read through her book, I can't help recognize the wealth of knowledge she presents, as well as the compassion she has for saving and healing the world."

—**Amelia "Mimi" Pohlman**, mother, wife, sister, daughter, friend, real estate mogul, production Assistant at SI and CNN, Sports Illustrated, MSG Networks, and New York Rangers Broadcast.

Printed in the USA
CPSIA information can be obtained
at www.ICGtesting.com
LVHW012250010224
770716LV00039B/1542